DIAGNOSIS OF CHOLECYSTOSES

DIAGNOSIS OF CHOLECYSTOSES

A radiological survey with clinical aspects

J.H.J. RUIJS M.D.   AND   S.G.Th. HULST M.D.
radiologist   internist

University Hospital Utrecht

1977

SPRINGER-SCIENCE+BUSINESS MEDIA, B.V.

ISBN 978-90-247-1932-7   ISBN 978-94-010-1059-7 (eBook)
DOI 10.1007/978-94-010-1059-7

FOREWORD

Cholecystoses, as dealt with in this book by Dr J. H. J. Ruijs, radiologist, and Dr S. G. Th. Hulst, internist, is an interesting clinical and pathological entity and is unique in that it was introduced into medicine by radiological examination.

Soon after the discovery of a usable contrast medium for the gallbladder examination – 35 years ago – some features of cholecystoses have appeared in publications: Rokitansky-Aschoff sinuses and adenomyomatosis.

Jutras' display at the Congress in Montreal in 1962, informed the international radiological world of the common basis for the many different manifestations of cholecystoses.

Every radiologist is now acquainted with cholecystoses, but as symptoms are sometimes extremely slight – radiological technique must be exact.

The aim of this book is to inform the clinician and surgeon on this clinical and radiodiagnostic entity, and to correlate symptoms and signs with the possible need for surgery. Drs Ruijs and Hulst have succeeded in presenting all this information clearly and succinctly.

C.B.A.J. Puijlaert, M.D.
Chairman and Professor
Department of Roentgendiagnosis,
State University Hospital, Utrecht

CONTENTS

INTRODUCTION

The group of gallbladder abnormalities called cholecystoses, consists of radiologically described entities in which pathogenetic factors are poorly understood and clinical aspects sometimes obscure.

Although the term 'cholecystoses' was not introduced by him, J.A. Jutras should be regarded as the initial introducer of degenerative gallbladder abnormalities. In his Hickey memorial lecture (33) he excellently documented the conditions which later became known as *hyperplastic cholecystoses*. These are abnormalities of the gallbladder wall which are primarily neither infectious nor neoplastic, but are the result of hyperplasia and degeneration of one or more structures of the wall.

This type of abnormality was already known under many different and sometimes confusing names. Jutras has been able to categorise them in a single pathogenetic nomenclature which has received general acceptance.

Jutras has not only promoted the radiological diagnosis, but he has also increased interest in gallbladder diagnostics in general. As a result the radiological symptomatology of the degenerative gallbladder abnormalities has become more and more comprehensive. Especially adenomyomatosis can manifest itself in a wide variety of ways in which signs – originally regarded as typical – are only partially present or even absent.

Clinical interest in these conditions was generally minimal and reported therapeutic successes – whether surgically or medically – have hardly been taken serious. Nevertheless it is at least worthwhile to know of and to look for these conditions and thereby broadening the field of gallbladder pathology from the clinical point of view.

Careful clinical evaluation may in due course elucidate more about these abnormalities which can only be of help to those patients with complaints indicating biliary tract disease in which no stones can be found. The dictum 'no stones, no biliary pathology' is – unhappily – too often the point of view of the clinician.

The scope of this book is to try to give an overview of the cholecystoses in which radiological as well as clinical aspects are summarized. All presented cases have been histologically verified. The diagnosis of cholecystoses does not require sophisticated techniques but only knowledge of the condition by the clinician and – in addition – an open eye of the radiologist.

ROENTGENDIAGNOSIS

I. THE NORMAL GALLBLADDER

I.1 Histopathological considerations

To make the radiological diagnosis of cholecystosis, an understanding of the normal macroscopic and microscopic anatomy and some functional aspects is important.

Macroscopically, the gallbladder is a small pear-shaped sack in which, normally, the bile secreted by the liver is concentrated and stored for subsequent participation in digestion.
Anatomically, the gallbladder can be subdivided into three parts:
- *fundus* which is the most distal third,
- *corpus* which includes the middle portion and
- *collum* or *infundibulum*, also called the *neck*, which is continuous with the cystic duct.

The cystic duct contains an internal spiral septum (spiral valve of Heister) and terminates in the common bile duct.

Microscopically, four layers can be distinguished in the wall of the gallbladder (fig. 1):
a. the *mucosa* which consists of a single layer of columnar epithelial cells arranged in small villi, also called plicae (folds) of the third order. These are arranged in larger folds, called plicae of the second order, which, in turn, are built up into plicae of the first order. The plicae of first and second order give the interior side of the gallbladder the appearance of a honeycomb.
  In the mucosa are very diminutive outpouchings known as the sinuses of Rokitansky-Aschoff, after their discoverers (6, 41). They are normally sparsely distributed and do not extend beyond the muscularis mucosae (40). These will subsequently be referred to as R.A.S. These sinuses are often confused with the crypts of Luschka which are supposed to be abberant bile ducts and also occur in the normal gallbladder wall (27).

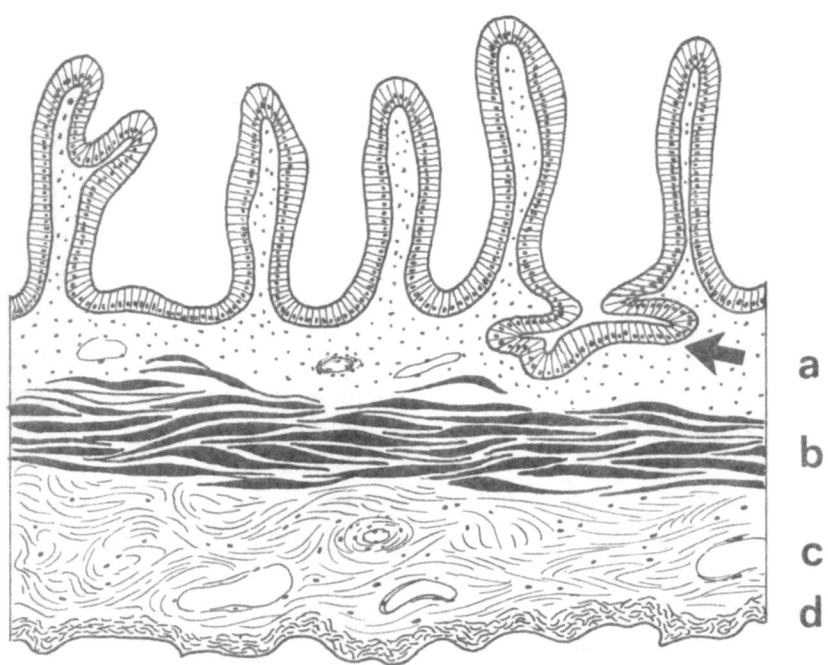

Fig. 1

Schematic representation of normal gallbladder wall.
a. Mucosa including subepithelium and Rotansky-Aschoff sinus (arrow).
b. Muscularis.
c. Perimuscularis.
d. Serosa.

The above mentioned structures sometimes take on a glandular aspect, but true glands do not occur in the gallbladder wall itself. However they can be found in the hepatic- and/or cystic ducts.

The gallbladder has no submucosa. A thin layer of loose connective tissue called the *subepithelium* lies directly under the mucosa and contains a system of fine capillaries.

b. The *muscularis* is chiefly a spirally arranged network of smooth muscular fibres.

c. The *perimuscularis* is sometimes known as lamina propria, lamina fibrosa or adventitia and consists of loose connective tissue containing capillaries, nerve fibres, and a few scattered leucocytes.

d. The *serosa* is continuous with the peritoneum and is thus absent where the gallbladder contacts the liver.

One must bear in mind that the total thickness of the gallbladder wall is about 1 mm, as this is important to the radiological differentiation of congenital septa and degenerative strictures.

Considering the functional aspects in diagnosing the cholecystoses it is important to bear in mind that the iodine containing contrastmedium – whether given orally or intravenously – reaches the liver via venous pathways and is then excreted into the gallbladder and mixed by the gallbladder with bile already present and concentrated. For a detailed analysis of this process may be referred to Berk and Loeb (8). Concentration is supposed to be a function of the mucosa.

In some pathological conditions such as chronic inflammation, neoplasm, and hyalinocalcinosis, reduced concentration can be caused by damage of the mucosa: none or poor opacification of the gallbladder occurs on the X-ray films. This is important in differentiating between these types of abnormalities from those in which the hyperplastic mucosa causes hyperconcentration of the contrast medium.

When the duodenal hormone cholecystokinin enters the blood by intravenous injection or after fatty food contraction-meal, the gallbladder contracts by virtue of the action of the muscularis.

In normal cases, a moderate volume reduction of approximately $^2/_3$ of the original diameter of the lumen is then visible radiographically.

In hyperplasia of the muscularis, the contraction can be increased from less than half the lumen to a complete evacuation of the gallbladder. This contraction is usually followed by the patient's experiencing an unpleasant feeling of discomfort, which sometimes is accelerated. This may be attributed to the neuromatosis which in many cases accompanies other forms of degeneration of the gallbladder wall.

II. THE CHOLECYSTOSES

II.1. Hyalinocalcinosis

Frequently referred to as 'porcelain gallbladder', 'calcified gallbladder' or 'calcifying cholecystitis', this condition is one of the most familiar of degenerative gallbladder wall conditions.

Histology
The lesion is based on hyperplasia of hyaline tissue in which calcium salts have been deposited. This process is accompanied by the loss of other normal structures present in the wall.

Roentgendiagnosis
Opacities due to calcium deposits with a typical 'shell' contour are visible on plain films of the gallbladder area. As a result of destruction of the mucosa, no concentration of contrast medium during cholecystography can occur in the gallbladder.

II/1.1. HYALINOCALCINOSIS (Porcelain gallbladder)

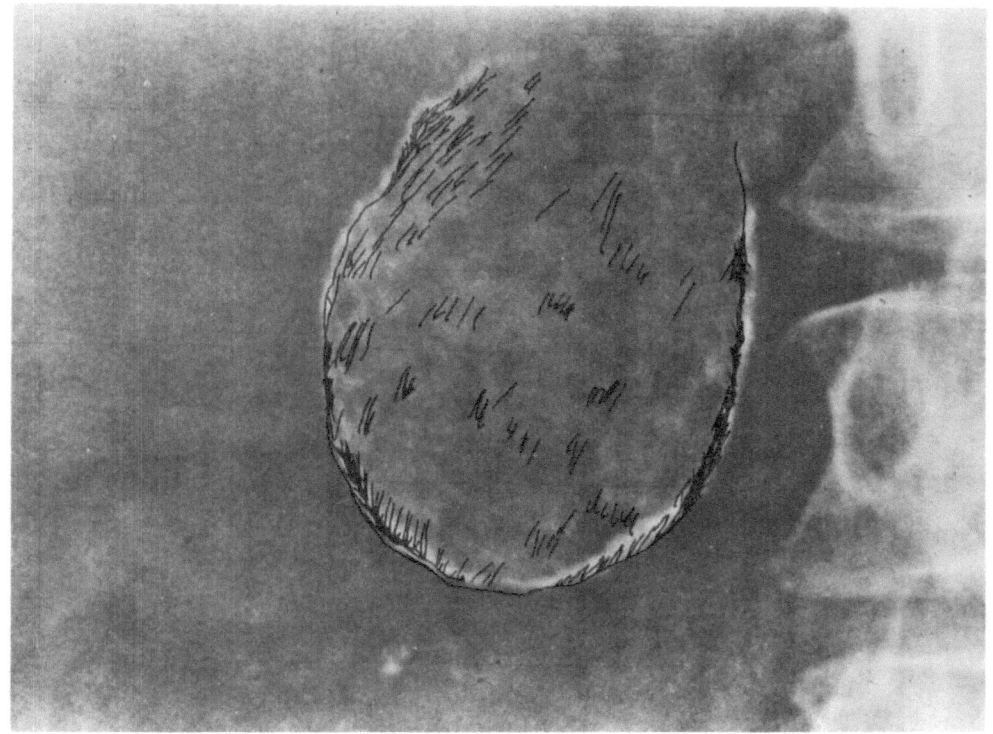

1. No function.
2. Calciumdeposits in the wall.

II.2. Cholesterolosis

Histology

Cholesterolosis is considered to be an accumulation of lipoid, chiefly in epithelial cells and histiocytes – 'foam cells' – coupled with epithelial hyperplasia. As a result, cholesterol-rich polypoid outgrowths of diverse shape and size develop (fig. 2). These may be solitary, multiple, or generalized – micronodular –. This last form has long been recognized by pathologists as 'strawberry gallbladder'.

Roentgendiagnosis

During cholecystography, fairly good concentration of the gallbladder is visible with multiple poorly defined translucencies of various size which remain constant in spite of different positions of the patient.

Administration of a contraction meal is not always necessary, but in some cases useful for demonstrating the fixed defects more clearly.

In differential diagnosis, solitary neoplastic or granulomatous polyps are sometimes difficult to distinguish from pseudopolyps. These two types of neoplastic growth are however very rare and, in most cases, the concentrating function of the mucosa is lost.

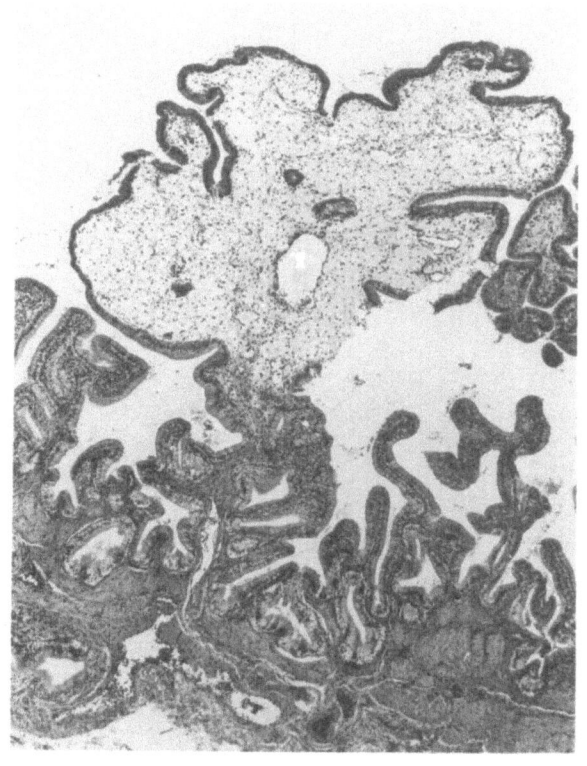

Fig. 2

Cholesterolosis of the gallbladder (detail): epithelial hyperplasia and pseudopolyp containing 'foam cells'.

II/2.1. CHOLESTEROLOSIS

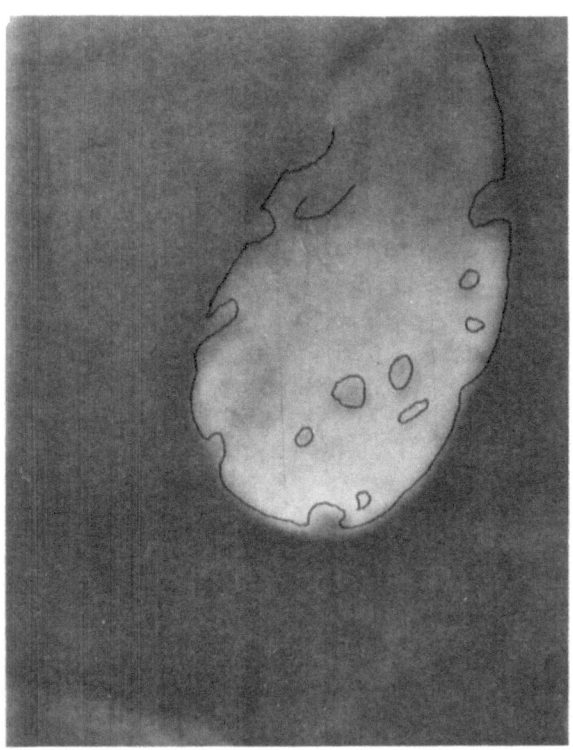

1. Fairly good concentration.
2. Multiple poorly defined translucencies.

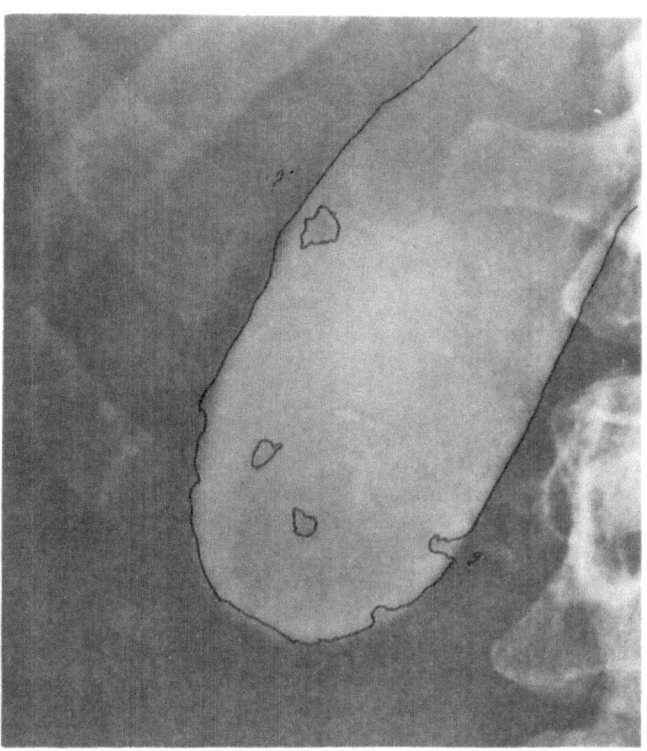

A 1. Fairly good concentration.
  2. Slight irregularities.
  3. Poorly defined
     translucencies.

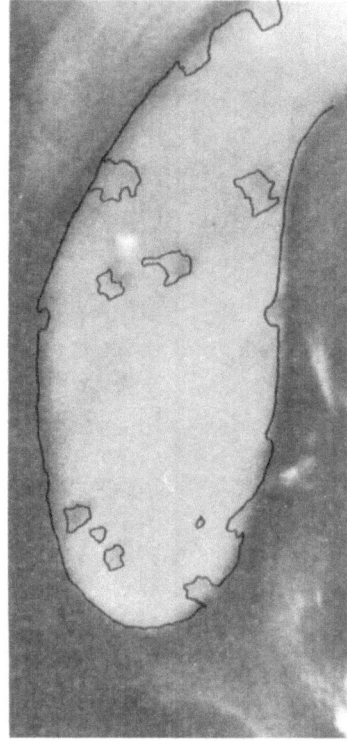

B After fatty meal:
  1. Good contraction
  2. More translucencies are
     visible now.

II/2.3. CHOLESTEROLOSIS

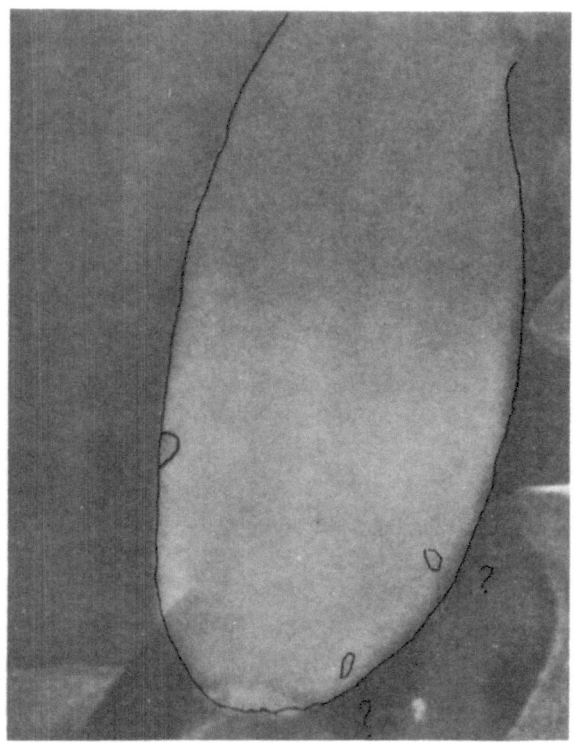

A 1. Good concentration.
2. Dubious translucencies.

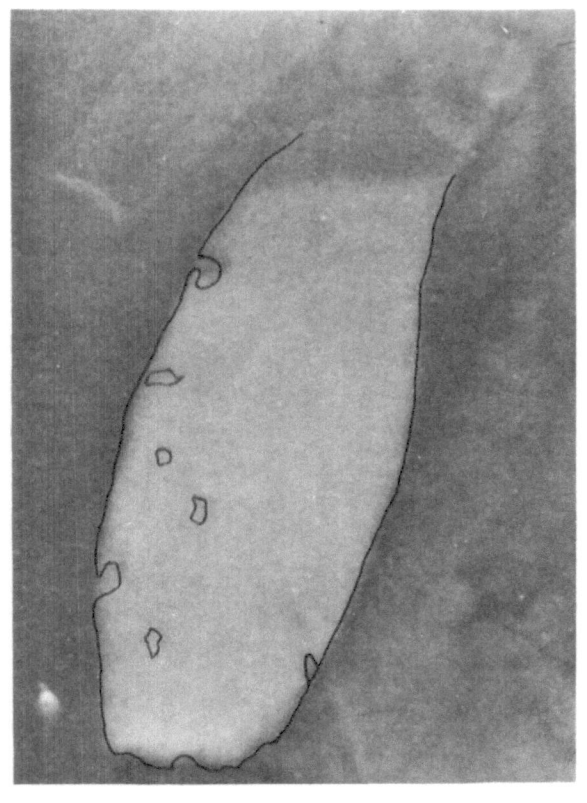

B After fatty meal:
Better visualisation of pseudo polyps

II/2.4. CHOLESTEROLOSIS (Local)

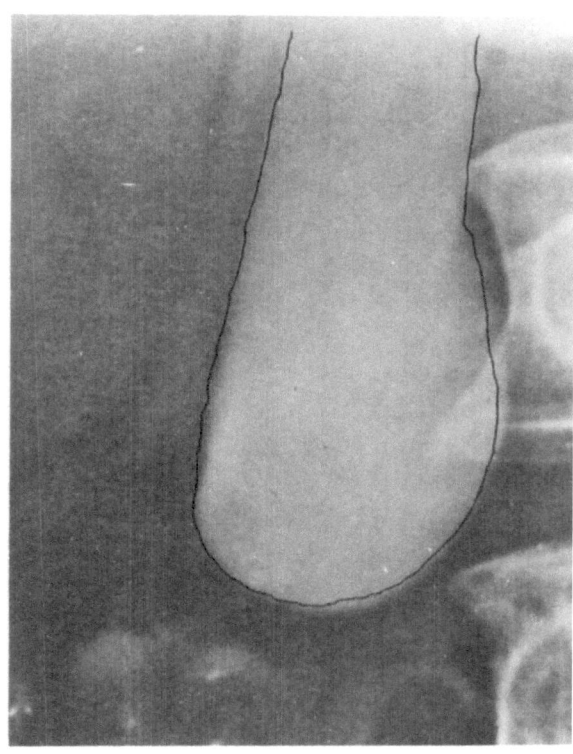

A 1. Good function.
2. "No abnormalities".

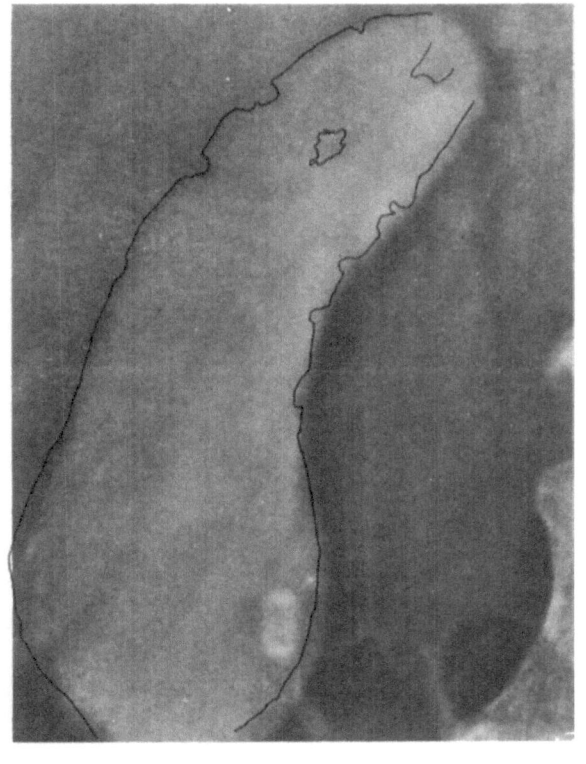

B Exposure with patient in supine position:
Multiple translucencies, mainly in the neck.

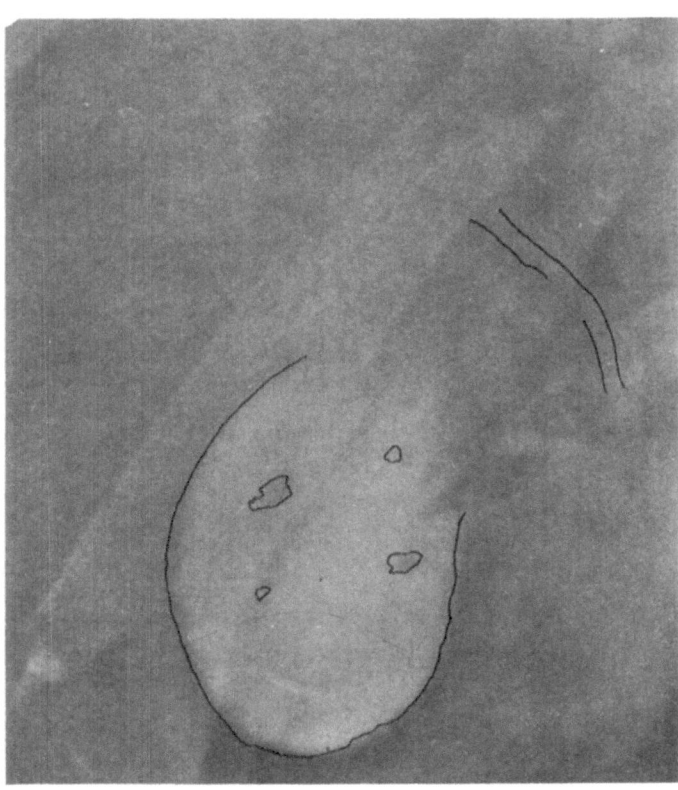

A Intravenous
  cholangiography:
  1. Good concentration.
  2. Multiple
     translucencies.

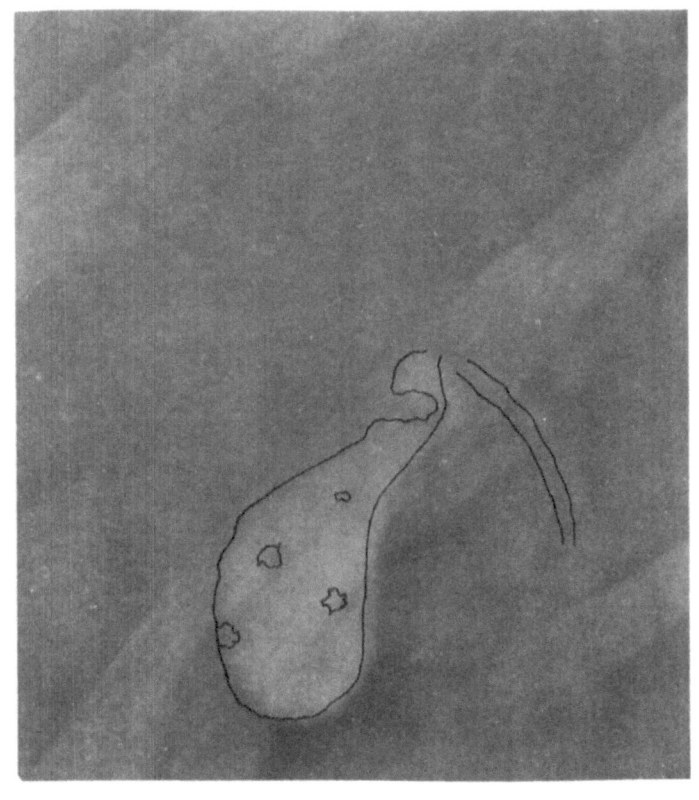

B After fatty meal:
  Hypercontraction of the
  gallbladder.

II.3. Adenomyomatosis

The term adenomyomatosis is used in cases of hyperplasia of the mucosa and muscularis. Since the publications of Jutras (33, 34) and Arianoff (4, 5), this type of gallbladder wall degeneration has gradually received more recognition.

Previously the deformities on the X-ray films were frequently described as 'congenital variations without pathological significance'. Terms such as 'hourglass gallbladder' (22, 23), 'fishhook gallbladder', 'bend', etc. exemplify this.

Histology
Microscopically, the mucosal hyperplasia manifests itself in a proliferation of the villi. The villi appear branched, giving rise to a pseudoglandular structure. The hyperplasia may also be distinguished by increase in size and number of Rokitansky-Aschoff sinuses. These push through weak places in the hyperplastic muscularis and remain in continuity with the lumen of the gallbladder (fig. 3, 4, 5).

This phenomenon is responsible for the synonymous name of 'intramural diverticulosis' (2, 12). The frequent coincidence of leucocytic infiltration in the surrounding tissue has given rise to the synonyms of 'cholecystitis glandularis proliferans' (36) and 'cholecystitis cystica' (35). Histologically there is often an association between this and other types of degeneration such as cholesterolosis, elastosis, lipomatosis, calcinosis, neuromatosis and fibrosis.

In the 'generalized' form of adenomyomatosis, the entire gallbladder wall is affected, but in the 'segmental' types only a portion of the gallbladder wall is involved. Some authors (1) divide these 'segmental' forms still further into proximal, middle and distal types.

From a radiodiagnostic point of view, subdivision of these various types of adenomyomatosis is not very worthwhile, as most of the 'localised' types are found to be more extensive on further radiodiagnostic and histological investigation than is to be first suspected. The 'localised' fundus type of Jutras (33) may be an exception in that it is identical with the well known 'adenomyoma' (11, 39, 44). Based on histological investigations, Jutras has demonstrated that 'adenomyoma', suggesting as it does a neoplastic condition with risk of malignant change, is a mistaken term as 'adenomyoma' is characterized by the same type of degeneration as adenomyomatosis.

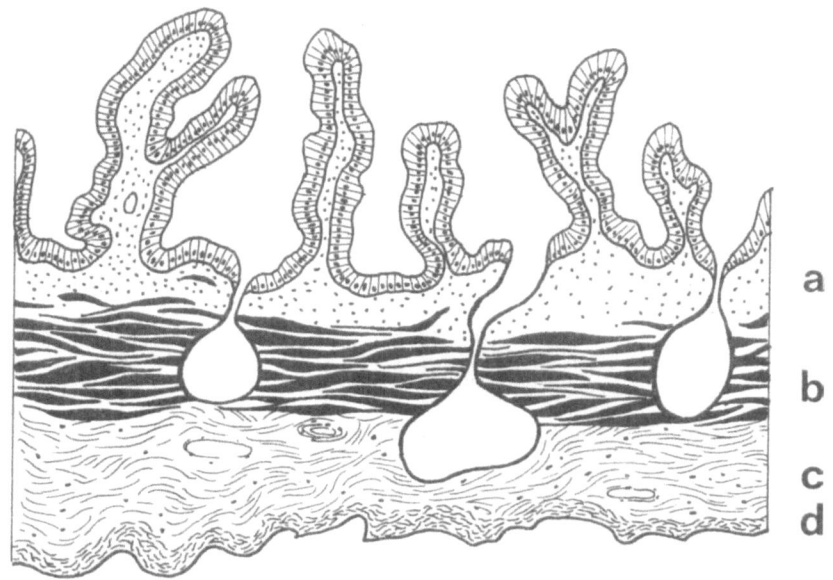

Fig. 3

Schematic representation of adenomyomatosis of the gallbladder.
a. Hyperplasia of the mucosa: the villi are more numerous and branched. More Rokitansky-Aschoff sinuses develop and they penetrate the muscularis.
b. Hyperplasia of the muscularis.
c. Perimuscularis.
d. Serosa.

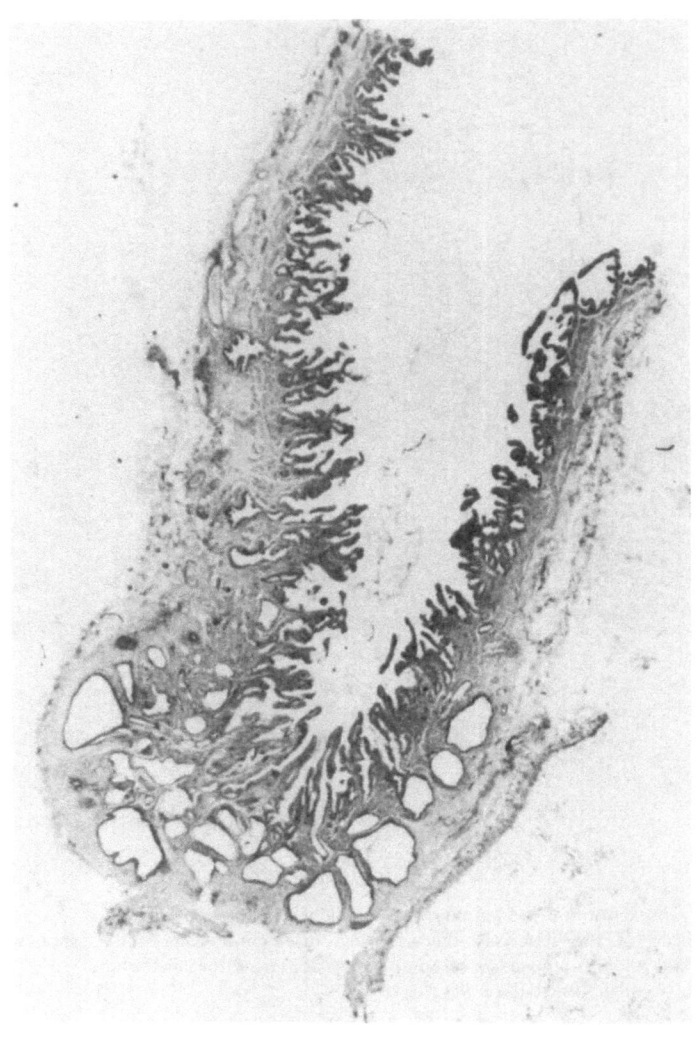

Fig. 4

Adenomyomatosis of the gallbladder: epithelial hyperplasia with R.A. sinuses chiefly in fundus area.

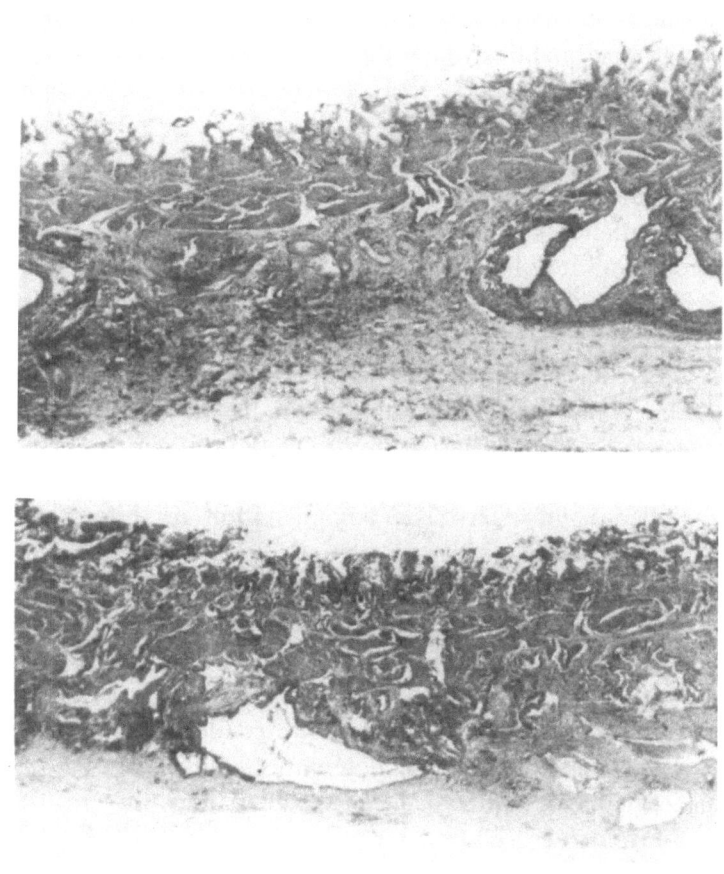

Fig. 5

Adenomyomatosis of the galbladder (details): epithelial hyperplasia with R.A. sinuses accompanied by muscular hyperplasia.

Roentgendiagnosis

In diagnosing adenomyomatosis, the greatest problem is the enormous variability of abnormalities which this condition can manifest (12, 19). Radiologically, two different characteristics allow the diagnosis of adenomyomatosis:

1. Indirect signs: These will be further discussed in Chapter IV. At this time, it is sufficient to mention that some of the 'indirect signs' such as hyperconcentration, hyperexcitation of hypercontractability, are often of great importance in supporting a diagnosis based on otherwise 'direct' signs.
2. Direct signs: These have been acknowledged by literature dating from 1948 (37). The most important sign is a demonstration of Rokitansky-Aschoff sinuses (R.A.S.). These are, during cholecystography observed to be fine opaque streaks and spots external to the contrastfilled gallbladder. The administration of a fatty meal is indispensable because after its administration the gallbladder contracts and more R.A.S. thereby become visible and appear more numerous. The distance between R.A.S. and the gallbladder lumen also increases as a result of the contraction of the hyperplastic muscularis.

   Not all Rokitansky-Aschoff sinuses are filled necessarily with contrastmedium as their connection with the lumen can be occluded by inspissated bile, microcalculi, or local inflammation.

In a large number of cases absolutely no filling of R.A.S. occurs, even after administration of a contraction meal. Attention must then be directed to other signs wich may be variable and are thus not all equally recognizable:

1. Deformities of the contour of the gallbladder, of which the best known are bandlike constrictions, 'shrivelling', 'hook' or spout-like deformation and sometimes other minor irregularities. It must be noted that these changes of the lumen occur in conjunction with a hyperfunctioning and an efficiently concentrating gallbladder.
2. Strictures: the presence of a stricture, or 'septum' on the X-ray films, is an important criterium for the diagnosis of adenomyomatosis. After administration of the contraction meal this 'septum' becomes shorter and thicker due to contraction of the hyperplastic muscularis. This

'septum' can easily be differentiated from a congenital septum which consists of merely a mucosal fold and therefore shows no contraction on the X-ray picture. Moreover, the total thickness of a congenital septum, as mentioned before, is not more than approximately 2 mm.

3. The combination of stones and a stricture is usually an indication of adenomyomatosis in the gallbladder wall. Where the gallbladder is 'shrivelled' with one or more stones impacted in the lumen, together with good function, diagnosis of adenomyomatosis can be established with certainty.

4. The combination of cholesterolosis with deformities and/or strictures is equally conclusive in diagnosing adenomyomatosis.

The localized fundus type, formerly known as 'adenomyoma', has a number of recognized typical forms of presentation. The criteria for diagnosis (1, 4, 5, 12, 33, 34) may be summed up as follows:

(a) a filling defect in the fundus of the contrastfilled gallbladder with:

(b) an opacity centrally in that defect and,

(c) occasionally R.A.S. visible surrounding the defect.

Demonstration of these abnormalities depends on their precise localisation in the fundus of the gallbladder by using multiple radiography views in different positions.

II/3.1. ADENOMYOMATOSIS

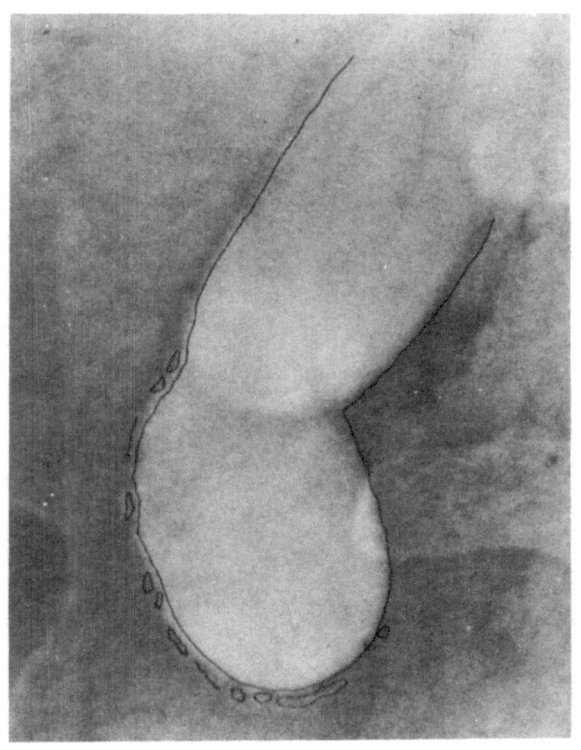

1. Good concentration.
2. Stricture in the middle of the corpus.
3. Contrast-filled Rokitansky-Aschoff Sinuses (R.A.S.).

II/3.2. ADENOMYOMATOSIS

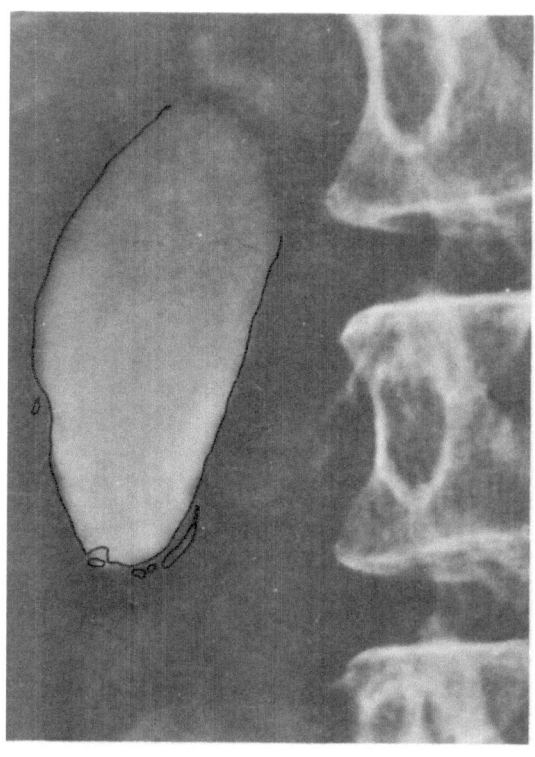

A 1. Good concentration.
   2. Rokitansky-Aschoff Sinuses (R.A.S.) visible.

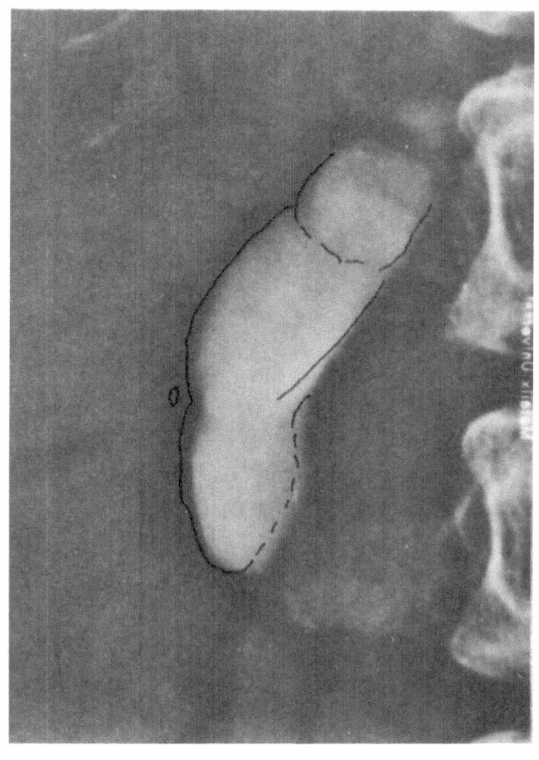

B After fatty meal:
   1. Hypercontraction.
   2. Strictures in the corpus.
   3. No better visualisation of R.A.S.

II/3.3. ADENOMYOMATOSIS (generalized form)

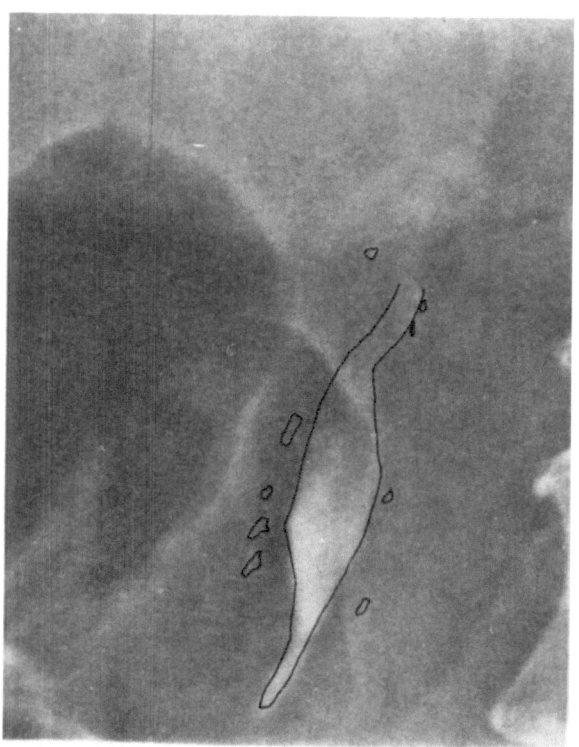

A 1. Good concentration with shrivelled and deformated lumen.
   2. Contrast filled R.A.S.

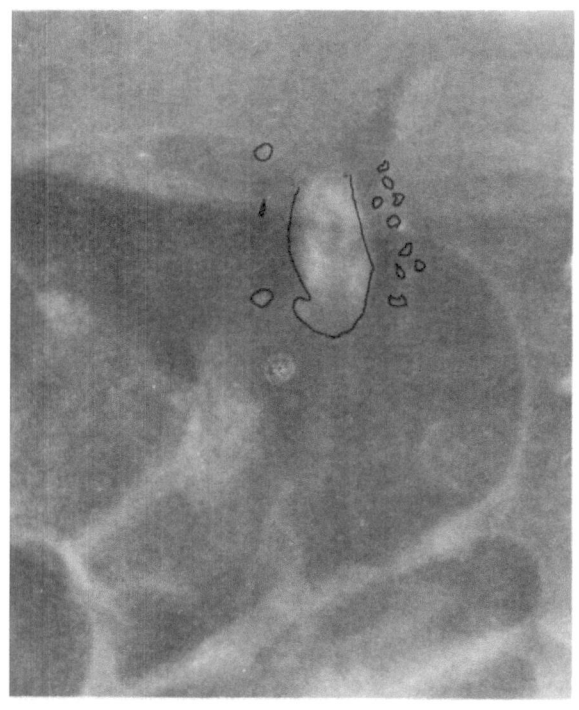

B After fatty meal:
   1. Hypercontraction associated with total evacuation of the fundus.
   2. Increased distance between R.A.S. and the lumen.
   3. Better visualisation of R.A.S.

II/3.4. ADENOMYOMATOSIS

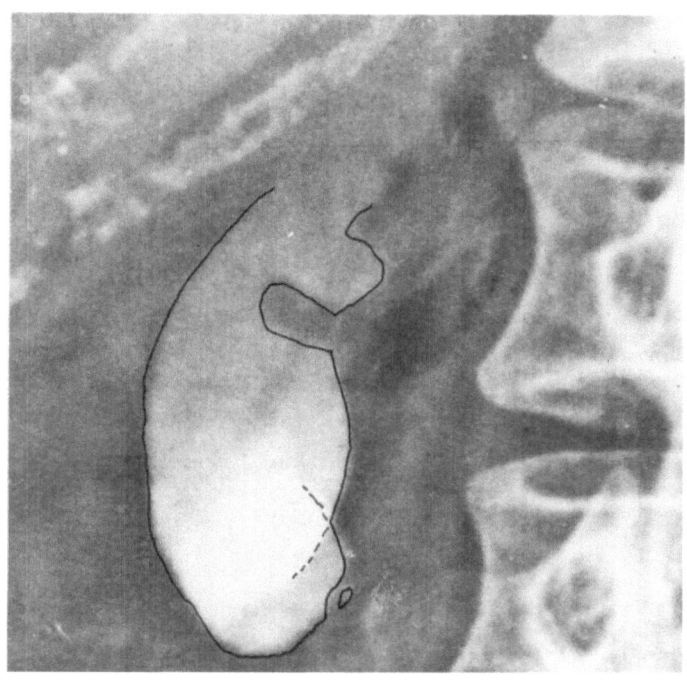

A 1. Good concentration.
2. Strictures.
3. Only one
   contrast-filled R.A.S.

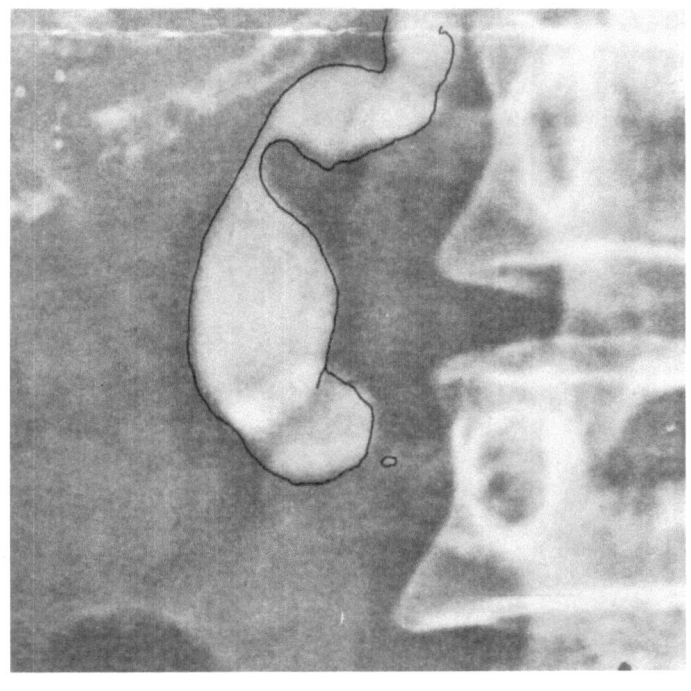

B After fatty meal:
1. Hypercontraction.
2. Contraction of the
   proximal stricture.
3. Increased distance
   between R.A.S. and
   lumen.

II/3.5. ADENOMYOMATOSIS (Generalized form)

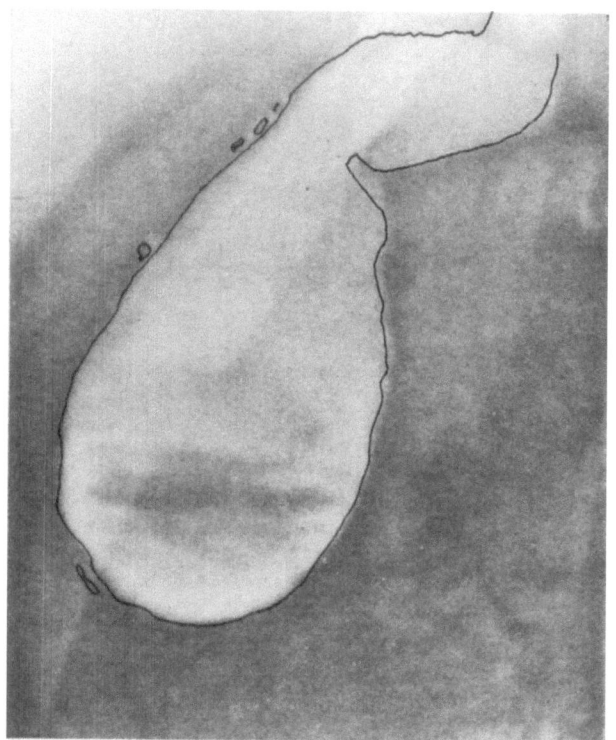

A 1. Good concentration.
2. Minimal deformities.
3. Stricture in the neck.
4. Few R.A.S. visible.

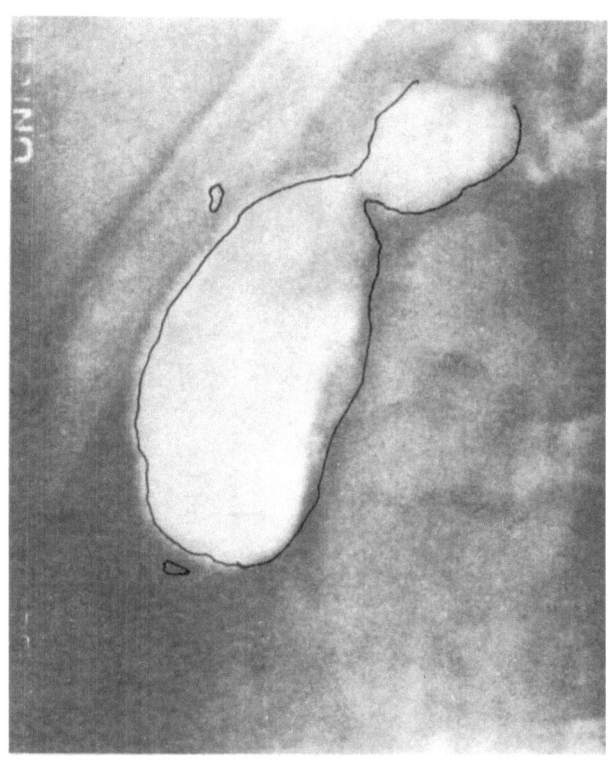

B After fatty meal:
1. Hypercontraction.
2. Contraction of the stricture.
3. Increased distance between R.A.S. and lumen.

II/3.6. ADENOMYOMATOSIS

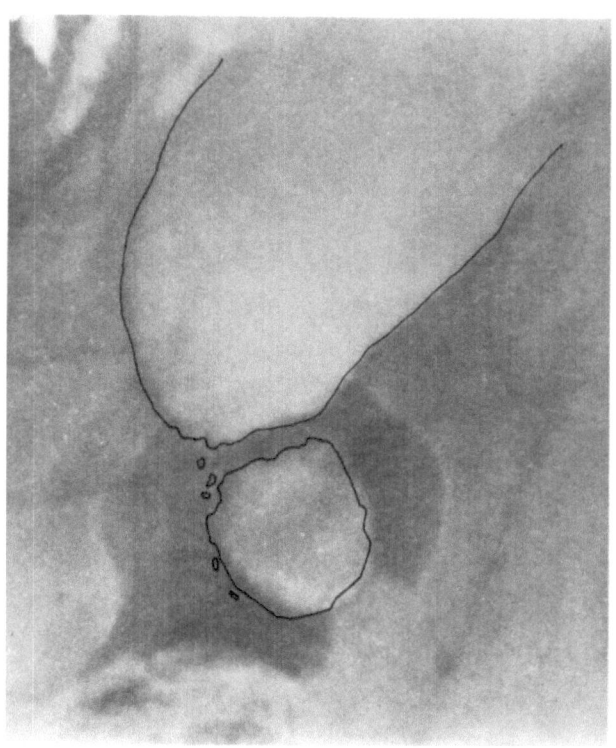

A 1. Good concentration.
   2. Stricture between corpus and fundus.
   3. Reduced volumen of distral third with
      slight irregularities.
   4. Few contrast-filled R.A.S.

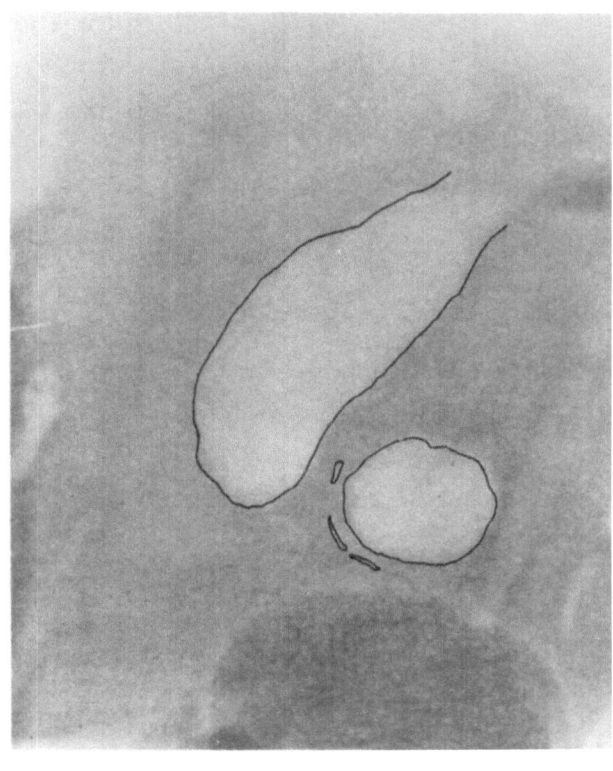

B After fatty meal:
   1. Hypercontraction.
   2. Contraction of the stricture.
   3. Better visualisation of R.A.S.

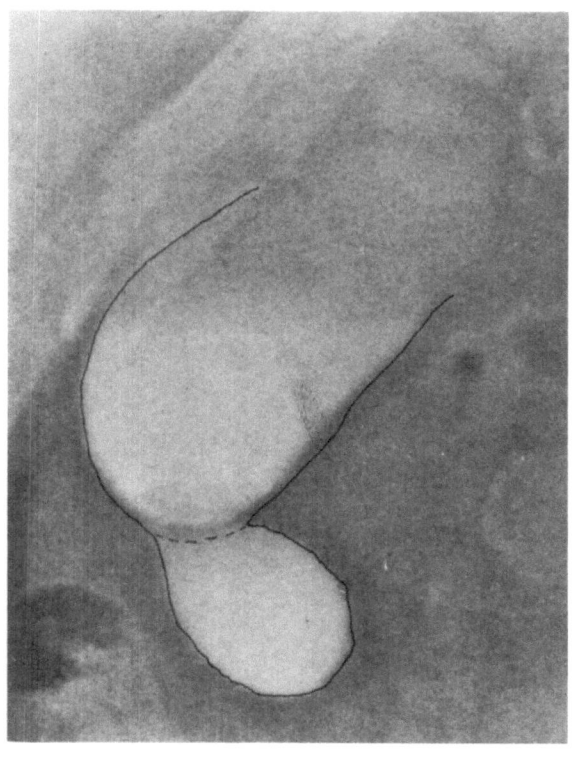

A 1. Good concentration.
   2. Stricture between corpus and fundus.
   3. Minimal irregularities in the fundus.
   4. No R.A.S. visible.

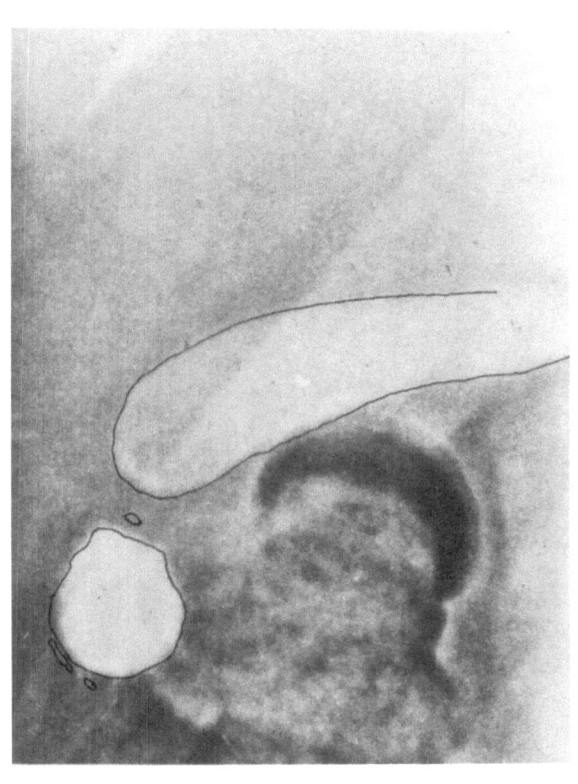

B After fatty meal:
   1. Hypercontraction.
   2. Contraction of the stricture.
   3. Filling of R.A.S. with contrast.

II/3.8. ADENOMYOMATOSIS

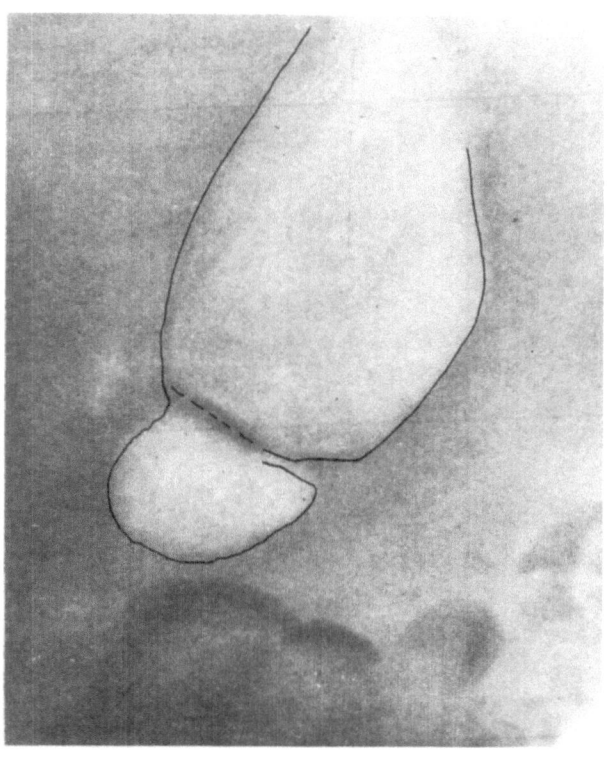

A (Magnified detail)
  1. Normal concentration.
  2. Stricture between corpus and fundus.
  3. No R.A.S. visible.

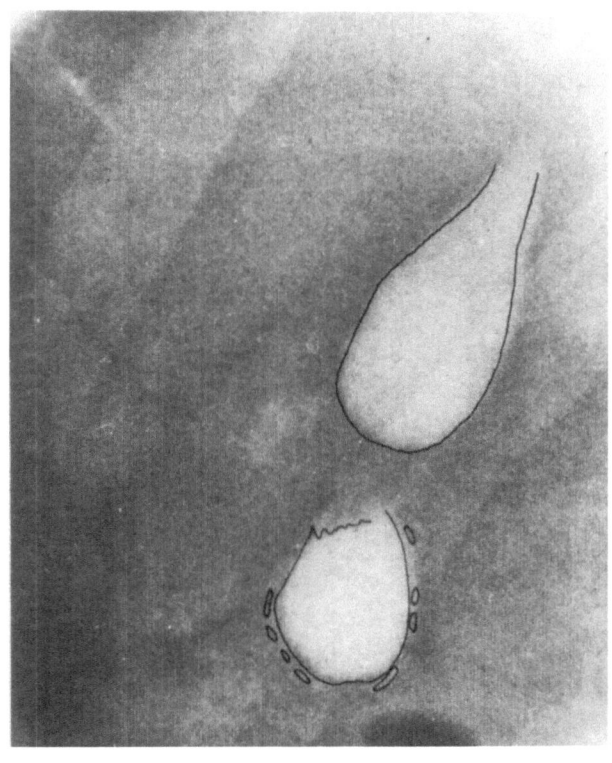

B (Magnified detail)
  After fatty meal:
  1. Hyperconcentration.
  2. Hypercontraction.
  3. Contraction of the stricture.
  4. Filling of R.A.S. with contrast.

II/3.9. ADENOMYOMATOSIS

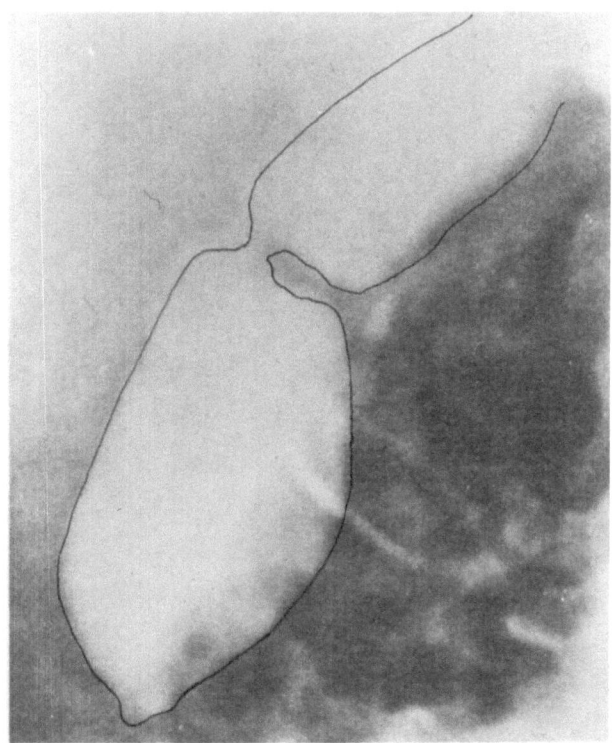

A 1. Minimal irregularities in fundus area.
2. Stricture between corpus and neck.

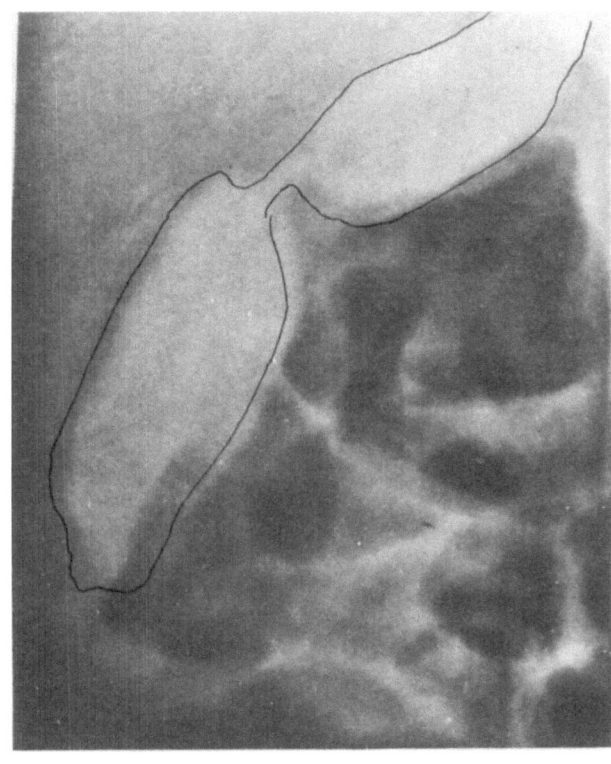

B After fatty meal:
1. Contraction of the stricture.
2. No R.A.S. visible.

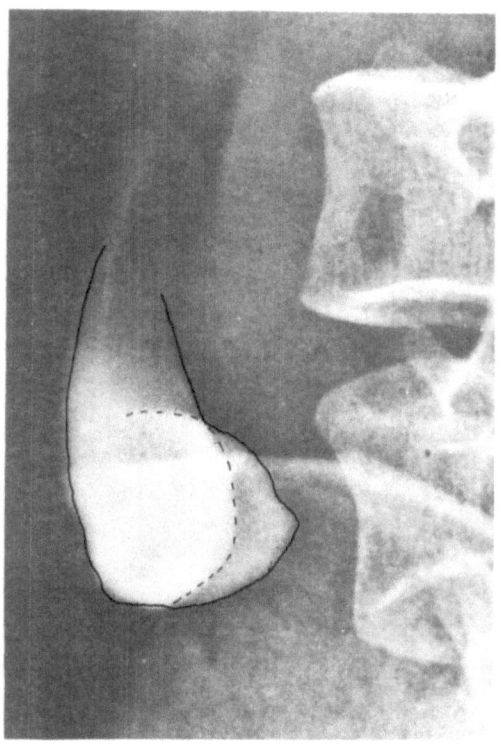

A Stricture between fundus and corpus.

B Spotfoto: Deformity of fundus.

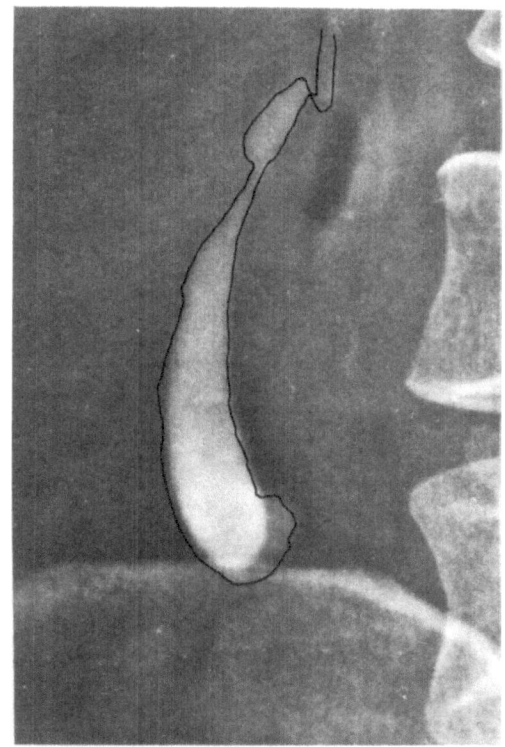

C After fatty meal:
  1. Hyperconcentration.
  2. Hypercontraction.
  3. No R.A.S. visible.

II/3.11. ADENOMYOMATOSIS

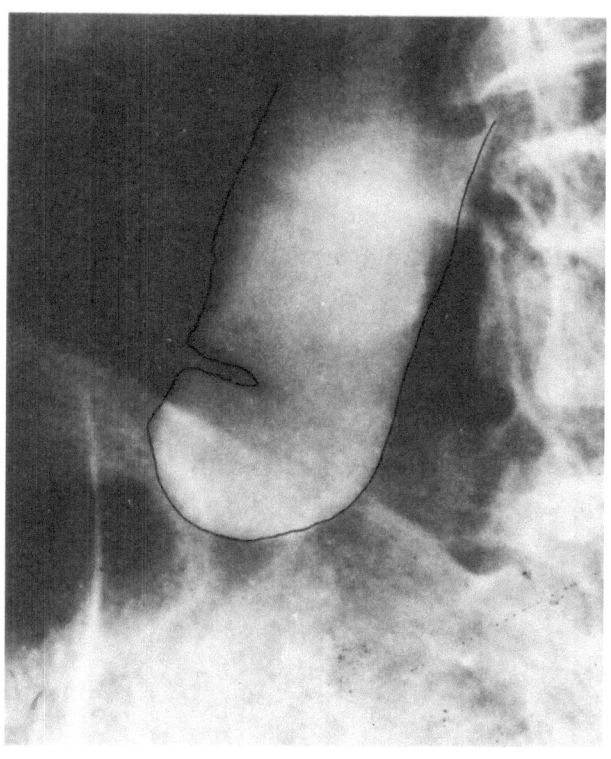

A Partial stricture between corpus and fundus.

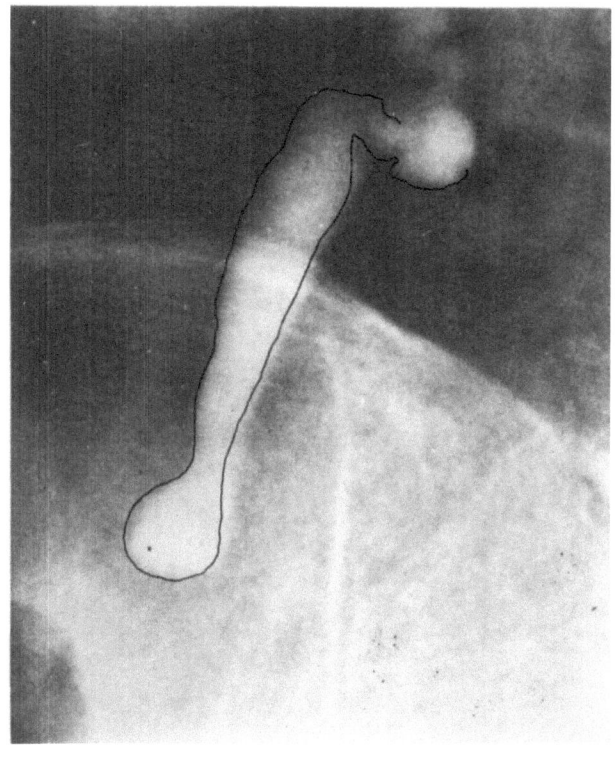

B After fatty meal:
1. Extreme contraction of the whole gallbladder.
2. Contraction of the stricture.
3. No R.A.S. visible.

II/3.12. ADENOMYOMATOSIS

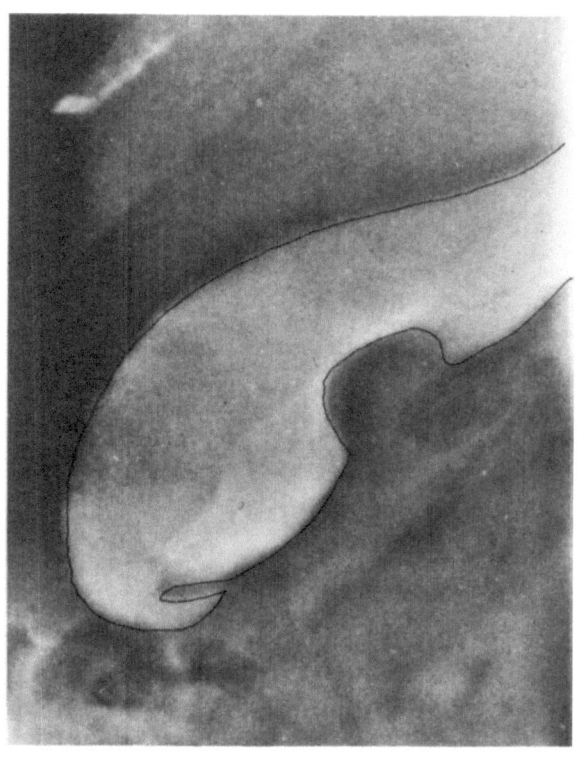

A Small stricture in
fundus area ('Fishhook')
(kinking between corpus and neck).

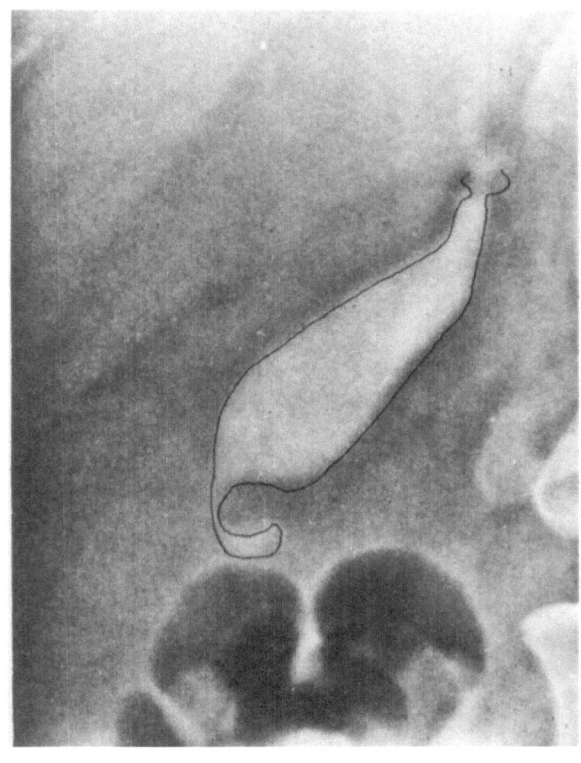

B After fatty meal :
1. Hypercontraction of distal part.
2. Contraction of the stricture.
3. No R.A.S. visible.

II/3.13. ADENOMYOMATOSIS

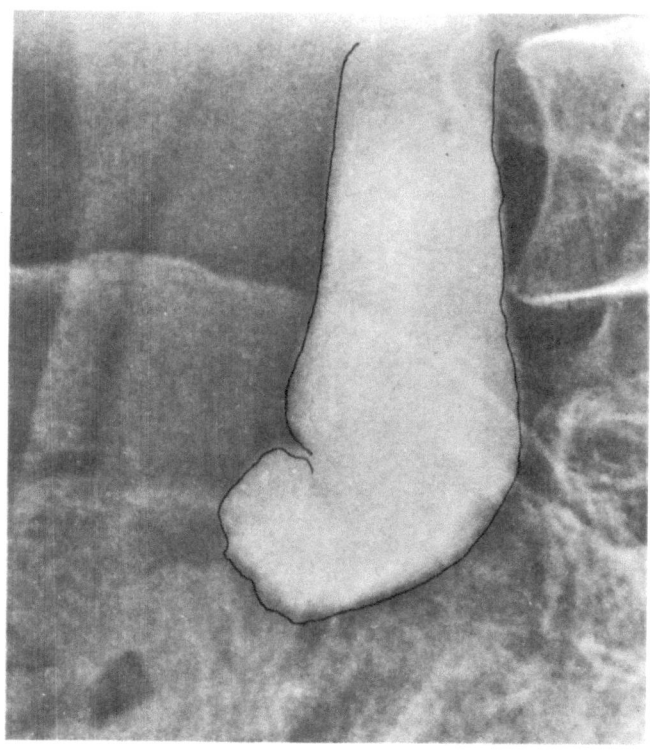

A 1. Small stricture between corpus and fundus.
2. Irregularities in fundus area.

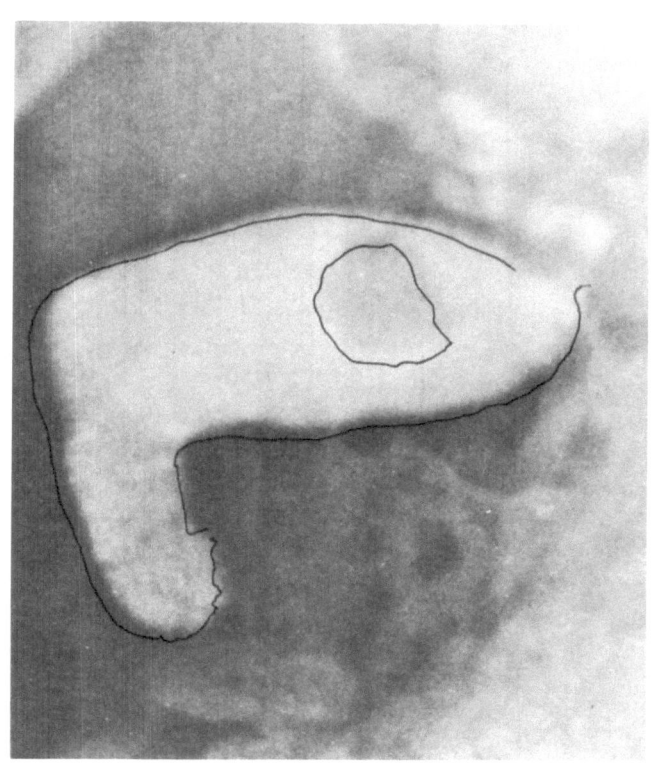

B After fatty meal:
1. Hypercontraction of distal part.
2. Poorly defined irregularities in fundus area (air bubble projected over collum).
3. No R.A.S. visible.

II/3.14. ADENOMYOMATOSIS

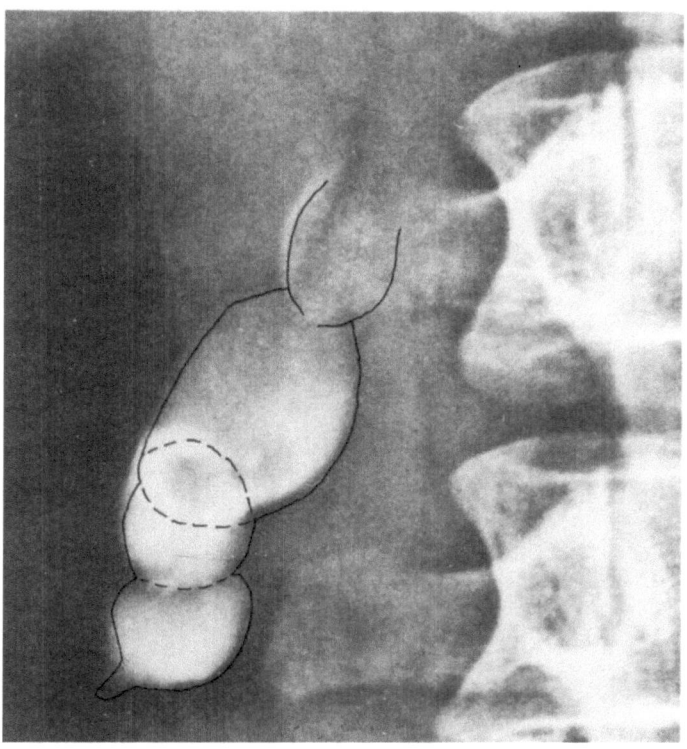

1. Stricture in corpus (airbubble overprojected).
2. Stricture between corpus and fundus.
3. Typical "spout" deformity of the distal part.
4. No R.A.S. visible.

II/3.15. ADENOMYOMATOSIS

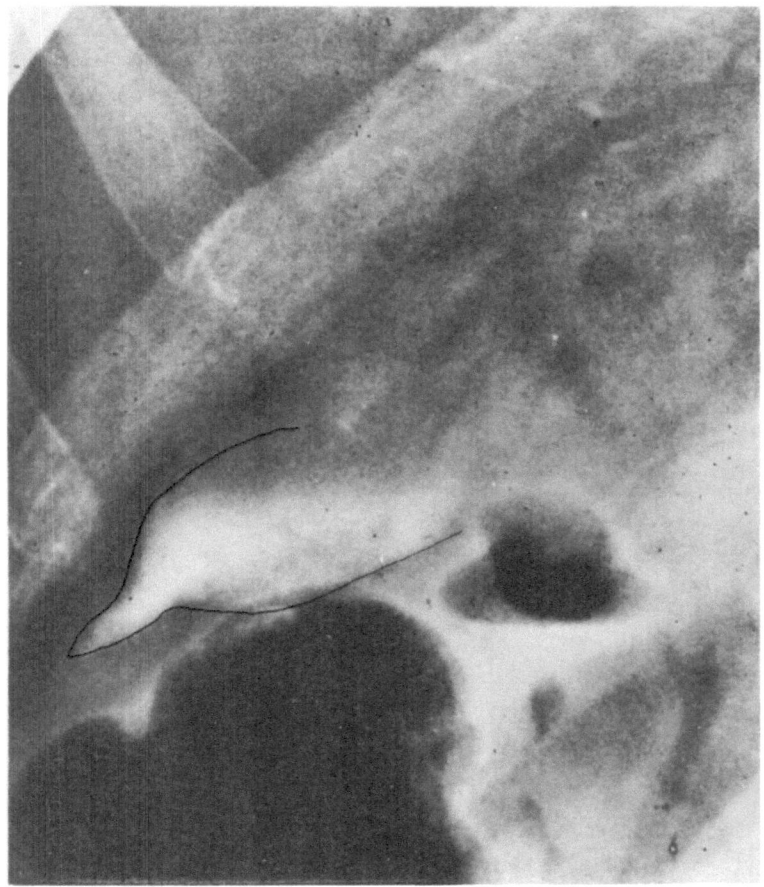

1. Small lumen.
2. Hyperconcentration.
3. Typical "spout" deformation distally.
4. No R.A.S. visible.

(This picture corresponds with fig. 4)

II/3.16. ADENOMYOMATOSIS (Segmental type)

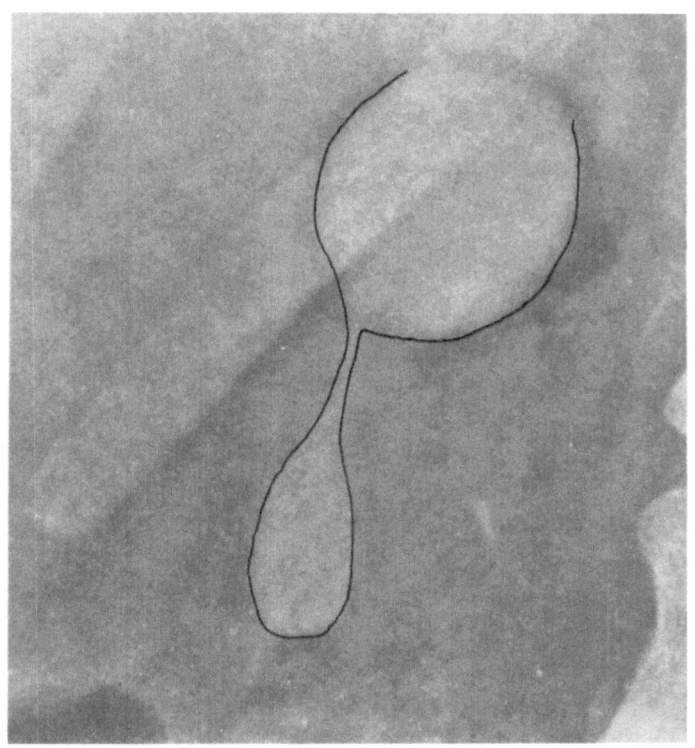

1. Good concentration.
2. "Shrivelling" in corpus and fundus area.
3. No R.A.S. visible.

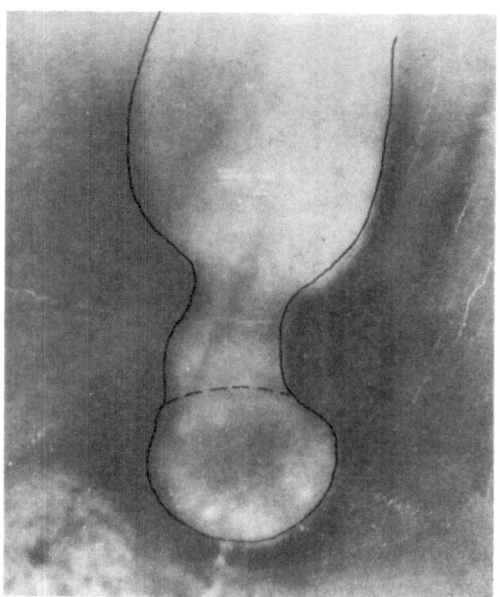

A "Shrivelling" of corpus.

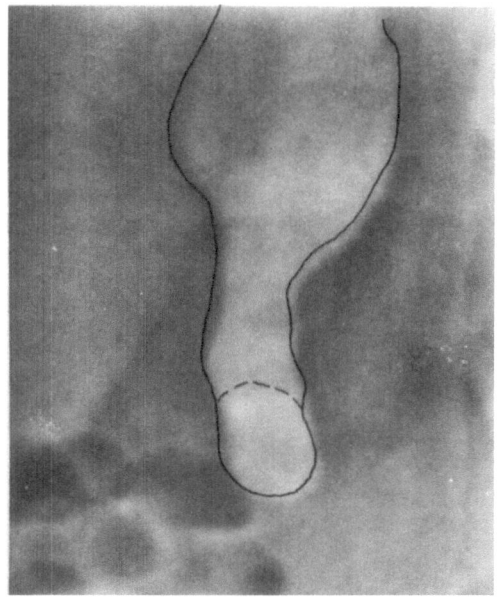

B The same gallbladder, four years later: Progression towards distal.

II/3.18. ADENOMYOMATOSIS AND CHOLELITHIASIS

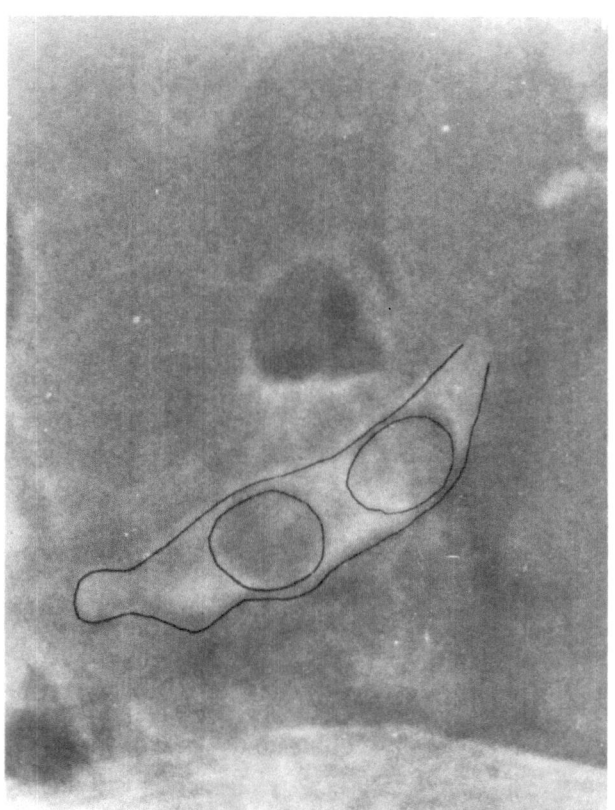

1. Good concentration.
2. "Shrivelled" lumen.
3. Irregularities in fundus area.
4. Two impacted stones.

II/3.19. ADENOMYOMATOSIS AND CHOLELITHIASIS

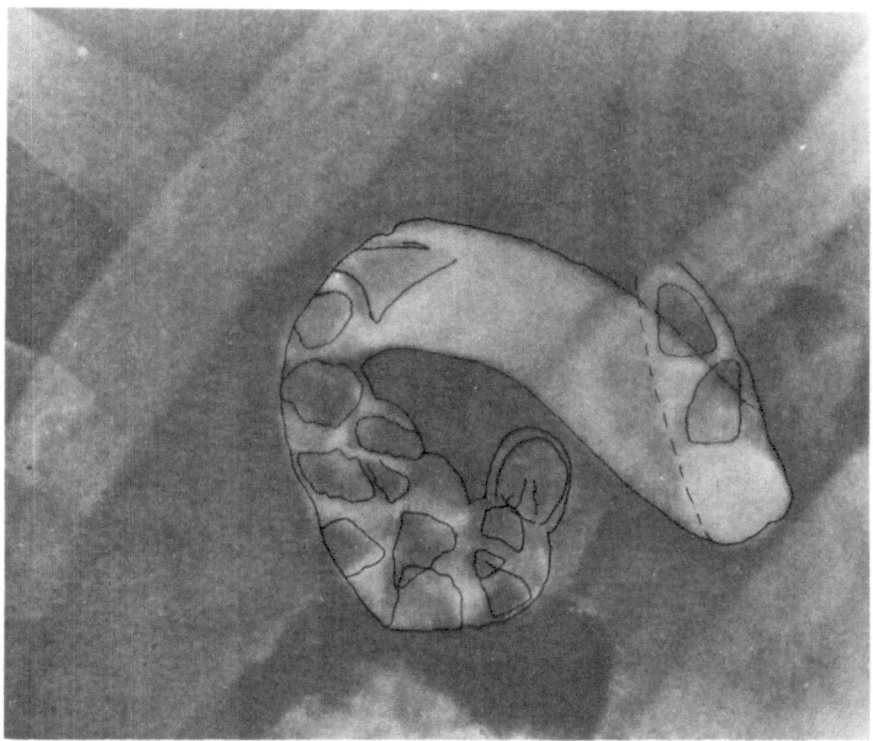

1. Good concentration.
2. Kinking and stricturation distally.
3. Stones in the lumen.
4. One stone impacted in the lumen of the fundus.

II/3.20. ADENOMYOMATOSIS AND CHOLELITHIASIS

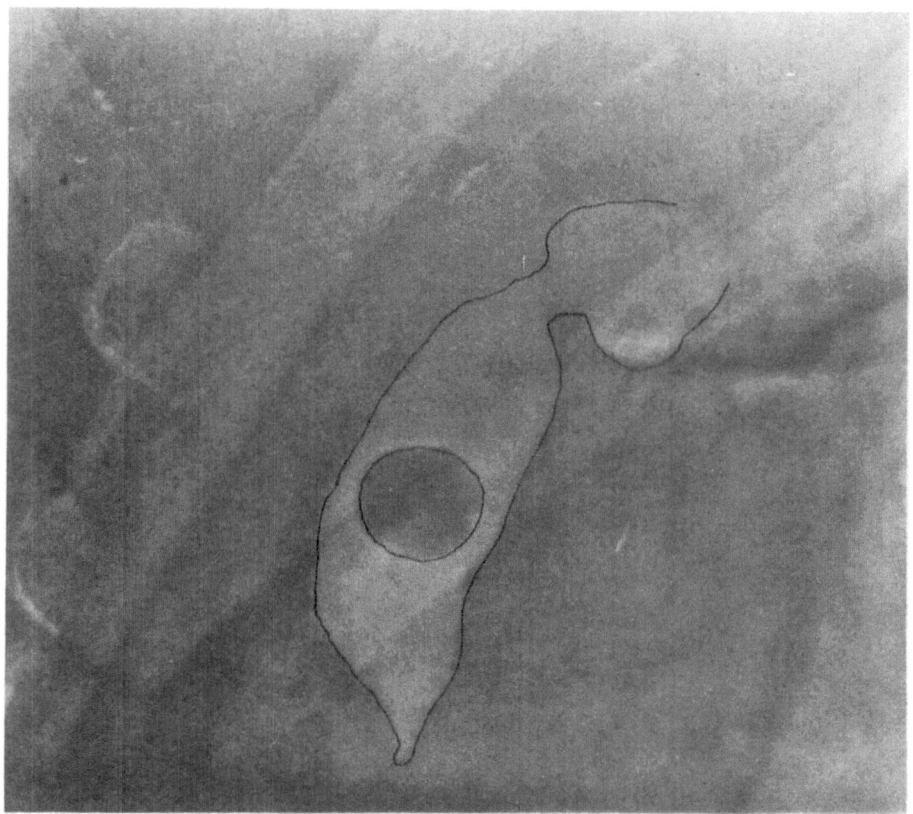

1. Stricture between corpus and neck.
2. Typical "spout" deformation distally.
3. One stone (not impacted).
4. No R.A.S. visible.

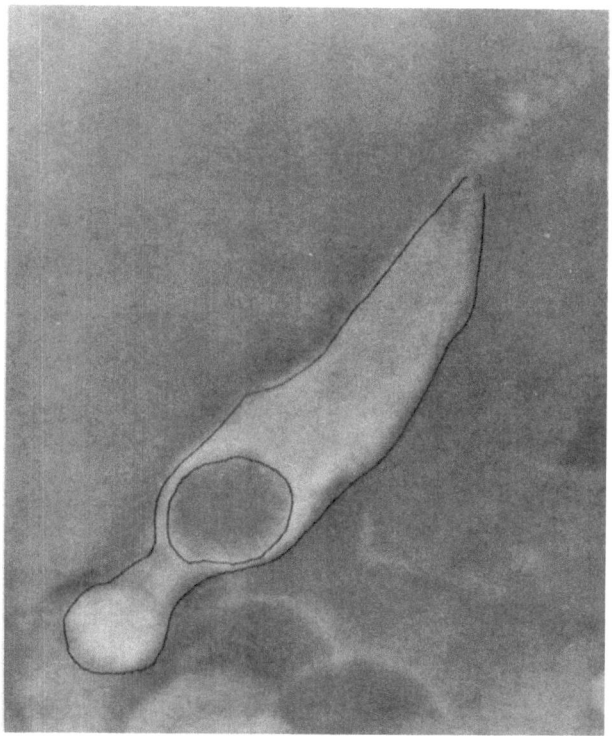

A 1. Good concentration.
2. Deformity of the distal third.
3. One stone (not impacted).

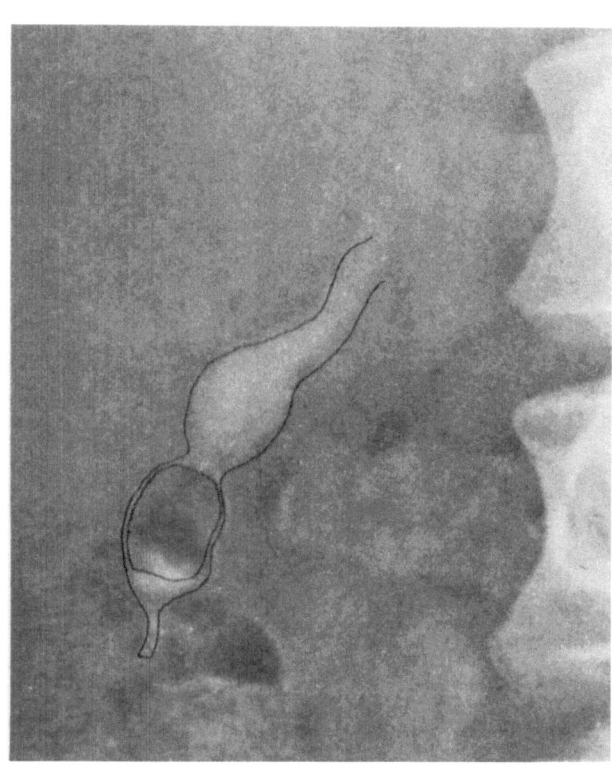

B After fatty meal:
1. Hyperconcentration.
2. Hypercontraction, associated with total evacuation of distal part and impacting of the stone.
3. No R.A.S. visible.

II/3.22. ADENOMYOMATOSIS AND CHOLELITHIASIS

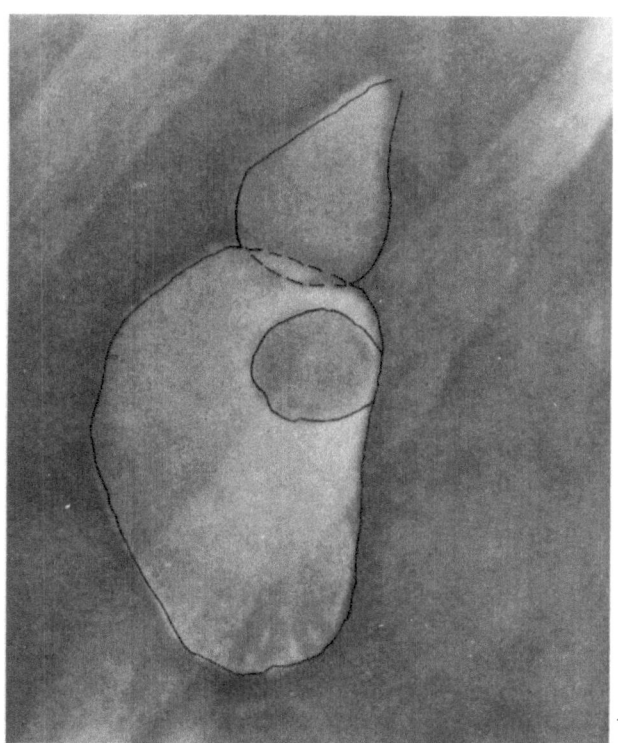

A 1. Stricture between corpus and collum.
  2. One stone.

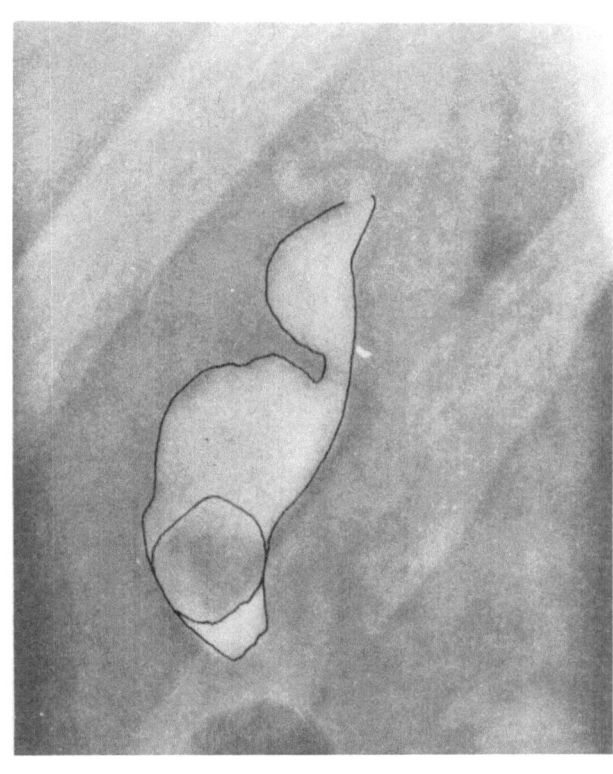

B. After fatty meal:
  1. Hyperconcentration.
  2. Hypercontraction.
  3. Contraction of the stricture.
  4. No R.A.S. visible.

II/3.23. ADENOMYOMATOSIS ASSOCIATED WITH CONGENITAL SEPTUM (Phrygian cap deformation) AND CHOLELITHIASIS

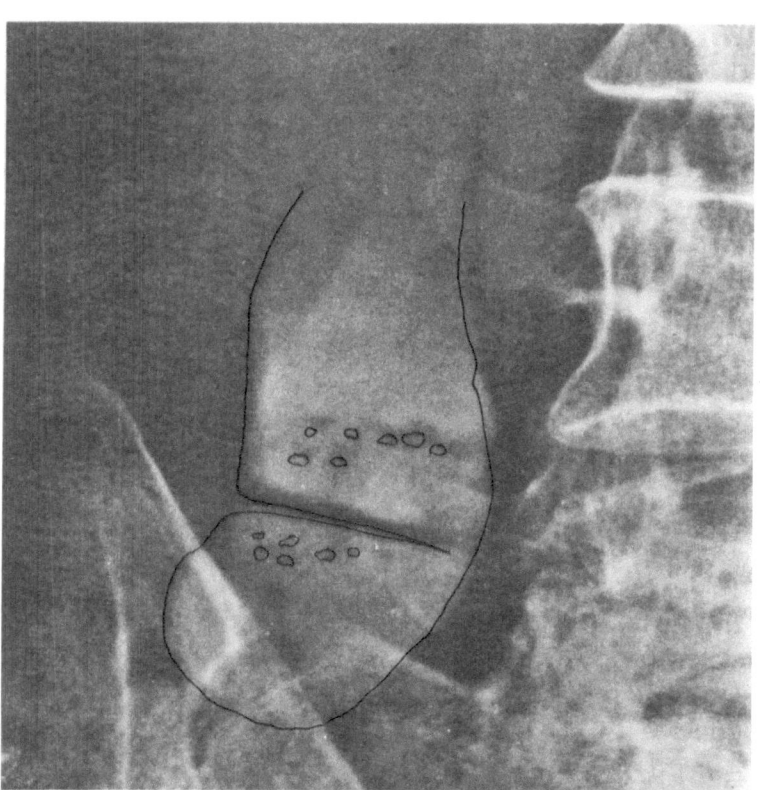

A (Exposure with the patient in erect position:)
1. Thin septum between corpus and fundus.
2. Translucencies in fundus and corpus.

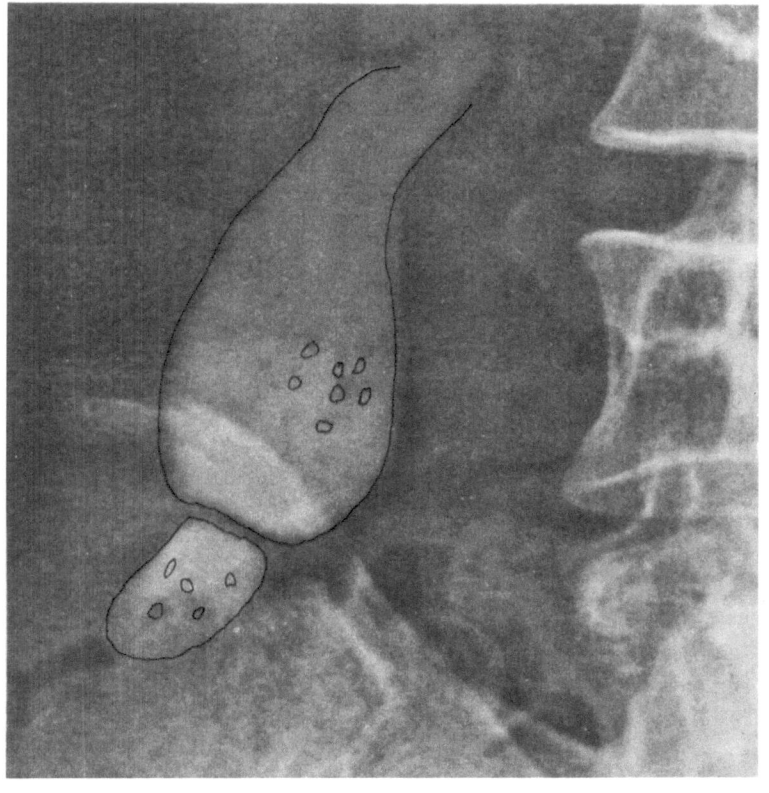

B After fatty meal: (Exposure with the patient in supine position:)
1. Hypercontraction of distal part.
2. No contraction of the septum.
3. Displacement of the translucencies.
4. No R.A.S. visible.

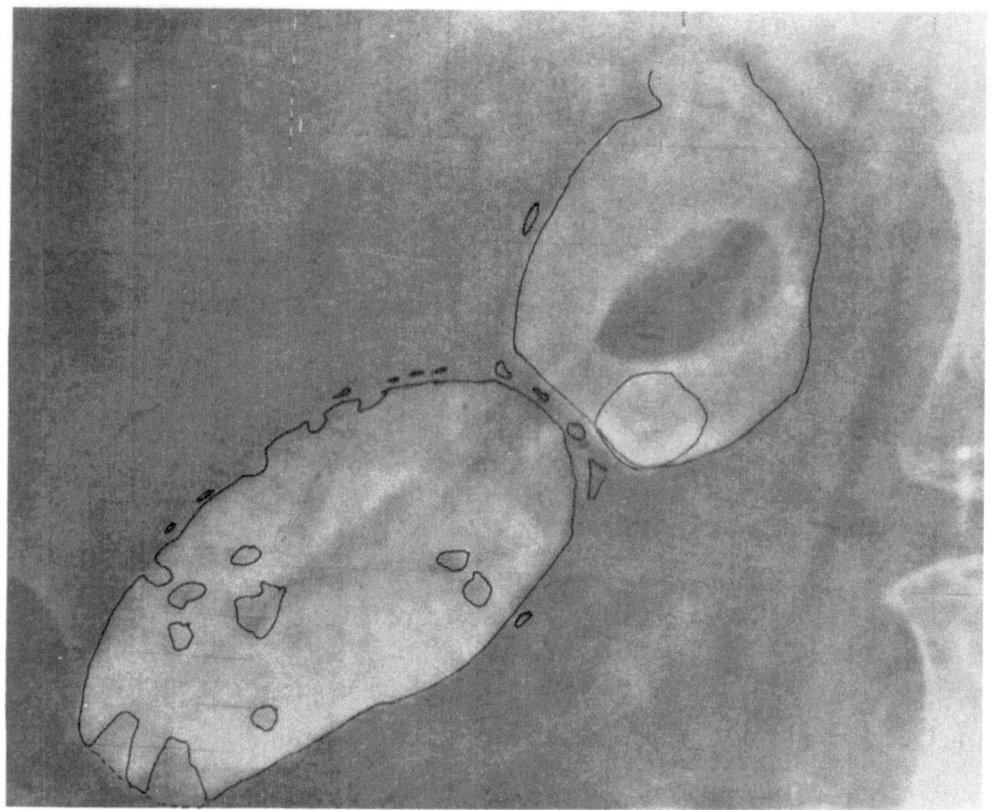

1. Stricture between corpus and collum.
2. Contrast filled R.A.S.
3. Pseudo polyposis.
4. One stone.

II/3.25. ADENOMYOMATOSIS (fundustype)

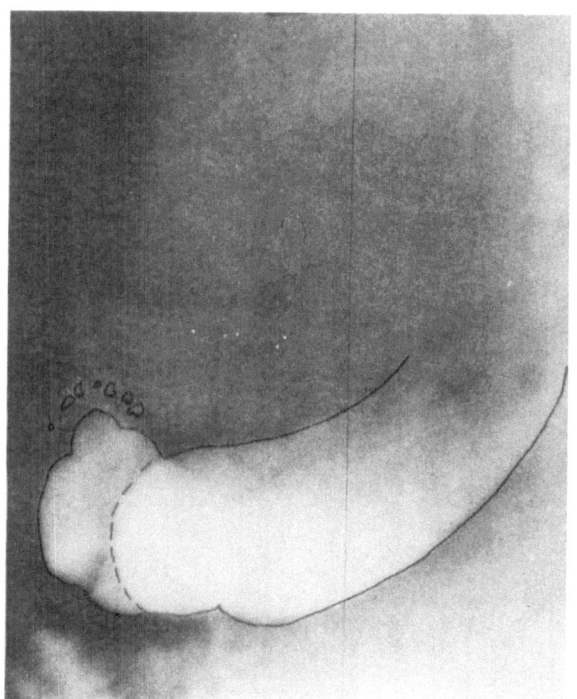

1. Defect in the fundus.
2. Contrast filled R.A.S. ("Rosette-sign")

II/3.26. ADENOMYOMATOSIS (fundus type)

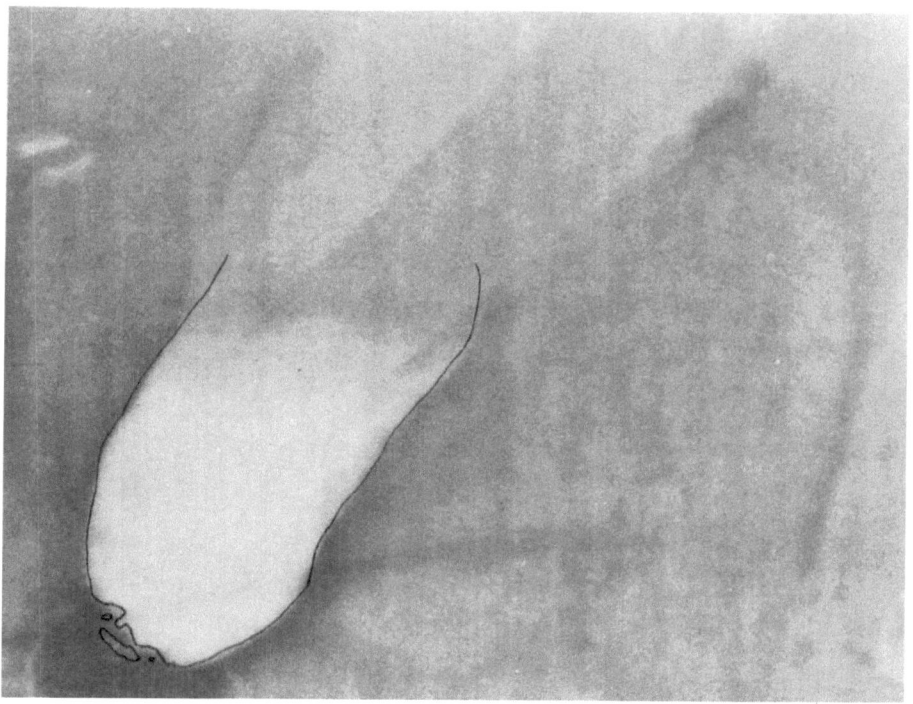

A 1. Good concentration.
2. Irregularities in the fundus area.
3. Contrast filled R.A.S.

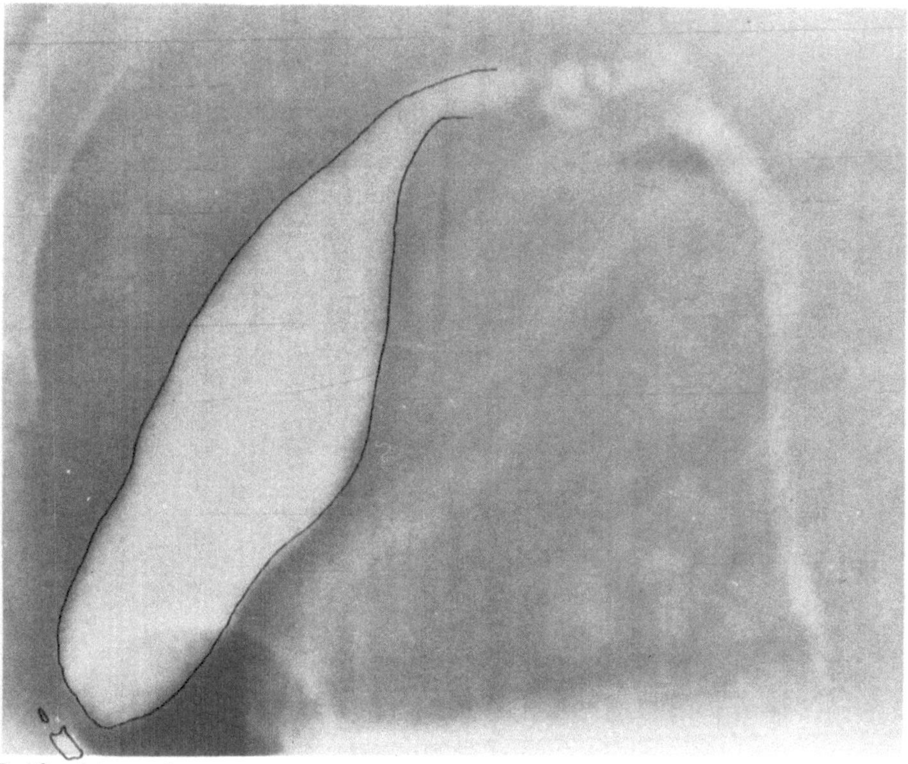

B After fatty meal:
1. Hypercontraction.
2. Increase of the distance between R.A.S. and the lumen.

II/3.27. ADENOMYOMATOSIS (fundus type)

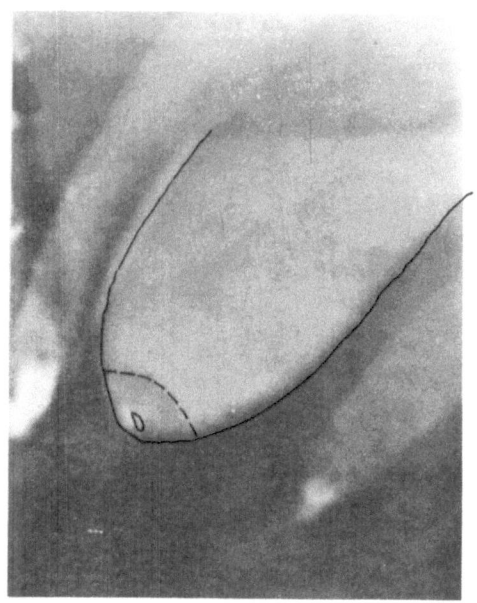

1. Typical defect in the fundus with an opacity centrally.
2. No R.A.S. visible.

II/3.28. ADENOMYOMATOSIS (fundus type)

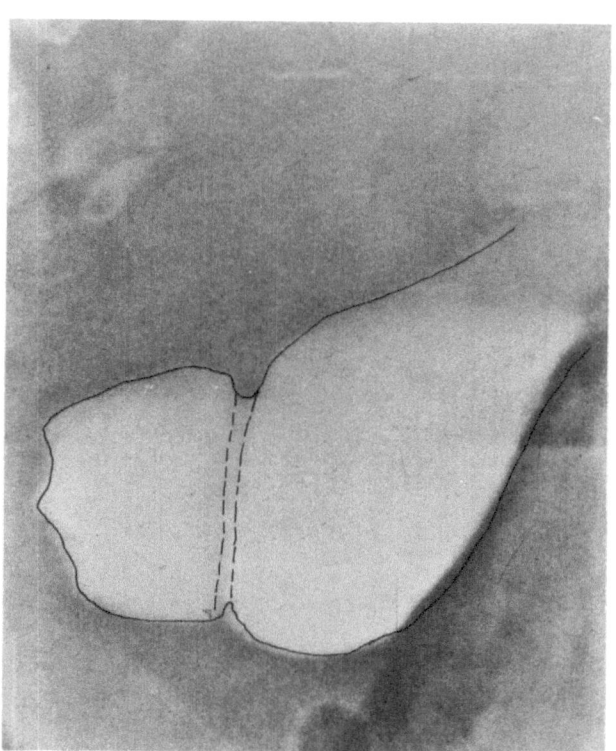

1. Stricture between corpus and fundus
2. Typical deformation of the fundus ("accolade-sign").
3. No R.A.S. visible.

II/3.29. ADENOMYOMATOSIS (fundus type)

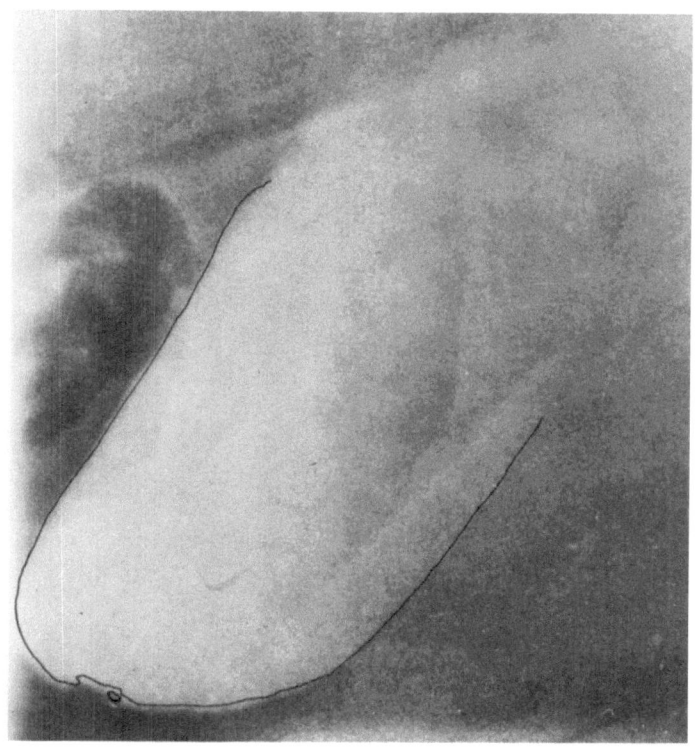

1. Minimal irregularity in fundus area.
2. One contrast filled R.A.S.

II/3.30. ADENOMYOMATOSIS (fundus type)

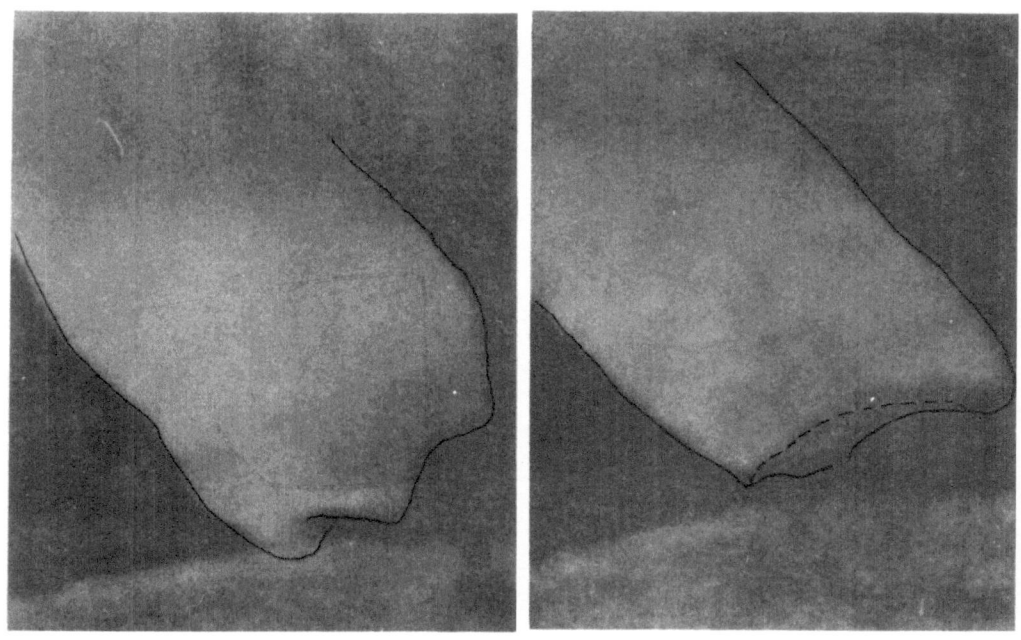

A "Accolade-sign".   B

A, B, C and D:
Four different views of the same type.

C   D

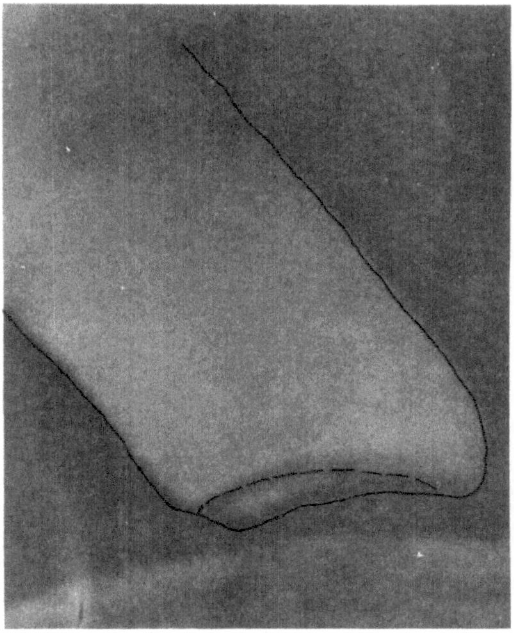

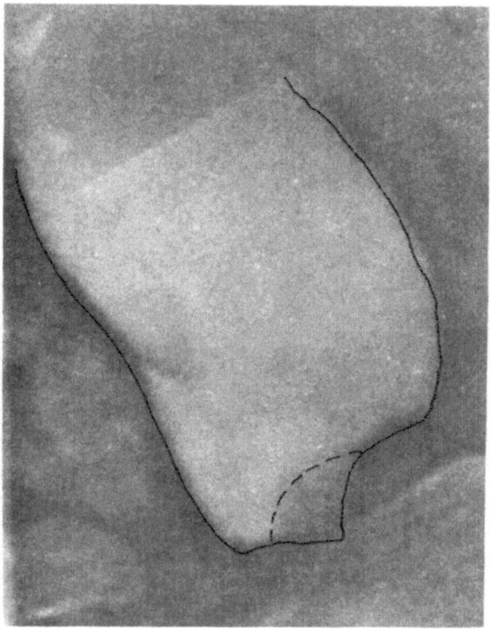

III. SOME DIFFERENTIAL DIAGNOSTIC PROBLEMS

III/1. DIFFERENTIAL DIAGNOSIS:

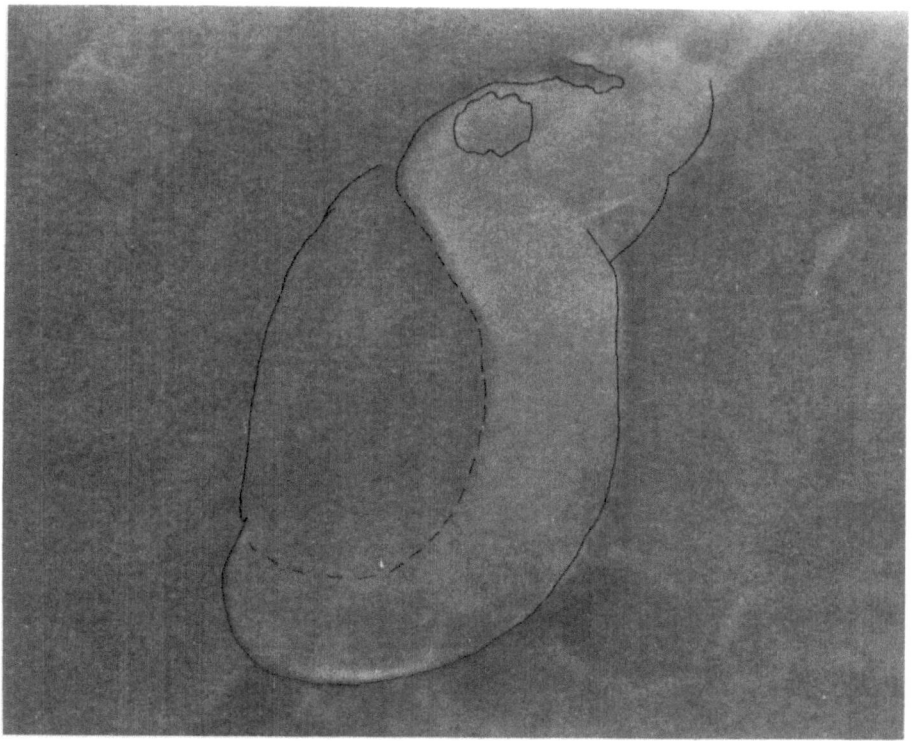

a. Cholesterolosis?
b. True polyp?
c. Stone?

1. Good concentration (with duodenal impression and kinking).
2. Translucency in collum which remains constant.

Discussion:
Follow-up studies and functional investigations are necessary.

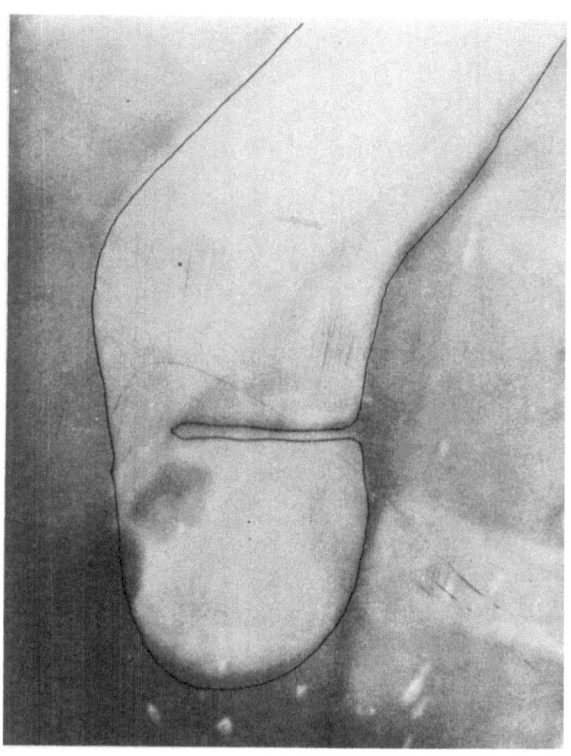

Gallbladder with thin 2 mm septum ("Phrygian Cap" deformation).

No adenomyomatosis.

III/3. ADENOMYOMATOSIS?

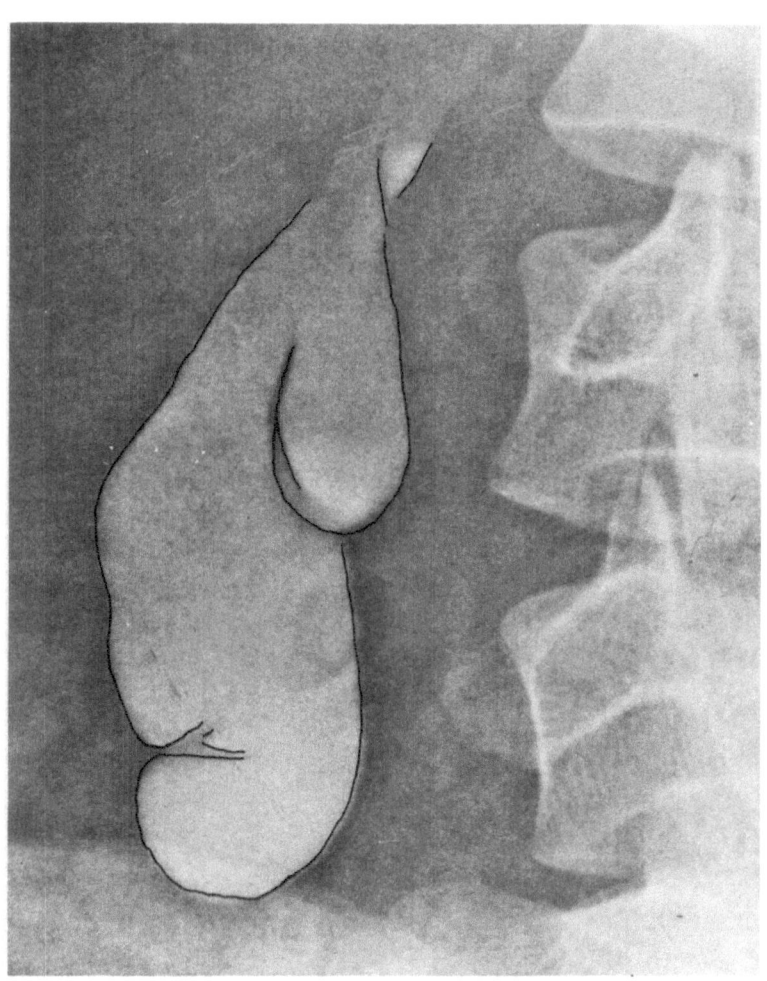

Two congenital mucosal folds.
No adenomyomatosis.

III/4. ADENOMYOMATOSIS?

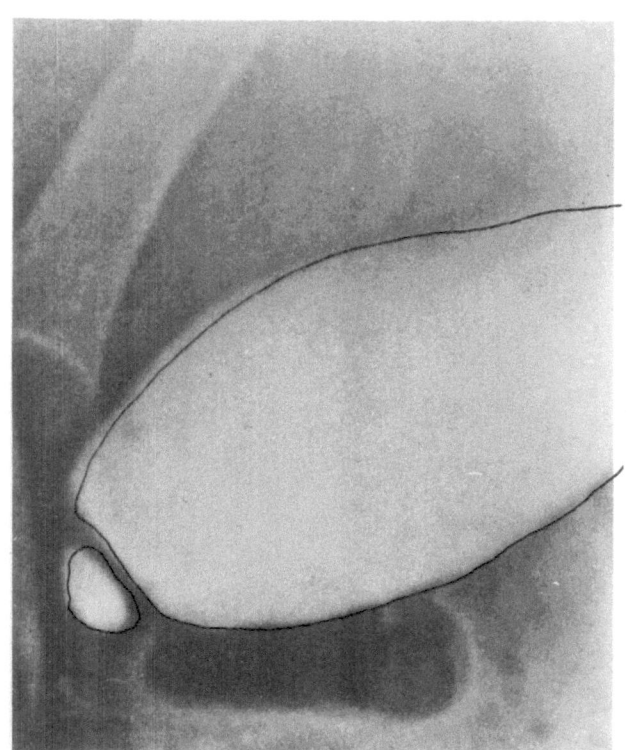

1. Stricture between corpus and fundus.
2. No R.A.S. visible.

Discussion:
functional investigation followed by
follow-up studies are necessary.

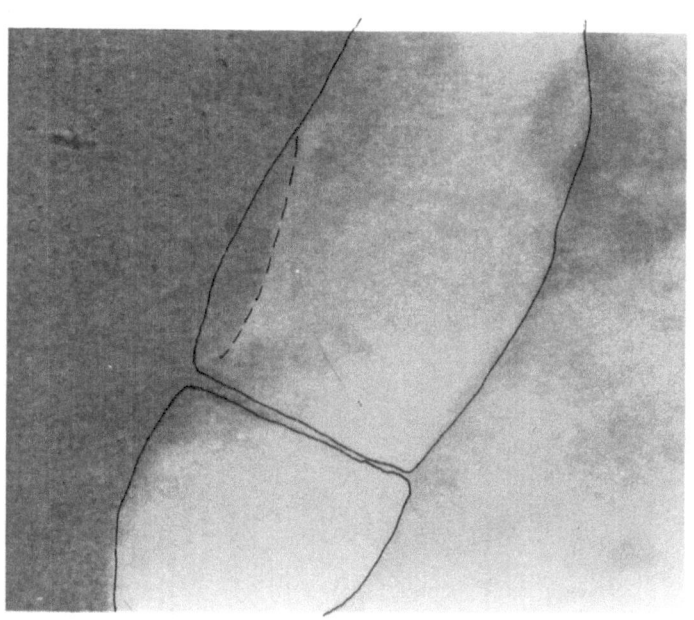

A Thin 2 mm-thick septum between corpus and fundus.

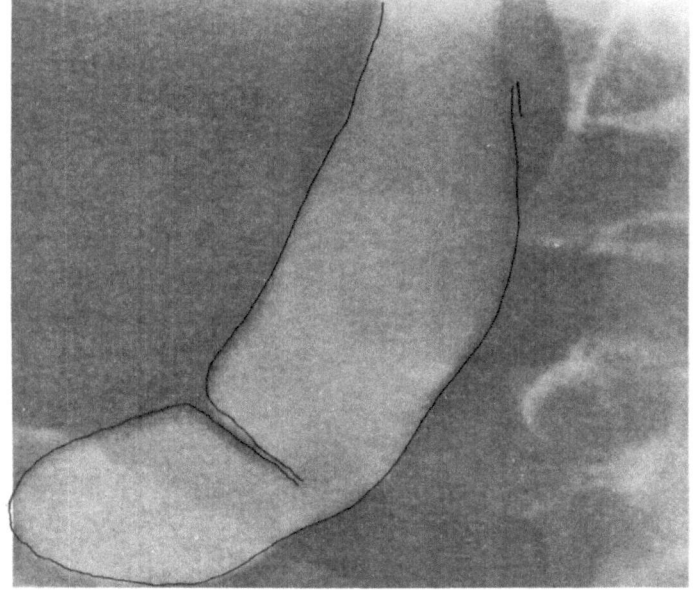

B After fatty meal:
1. Moderate contraction.
2. No contraction of the septum.

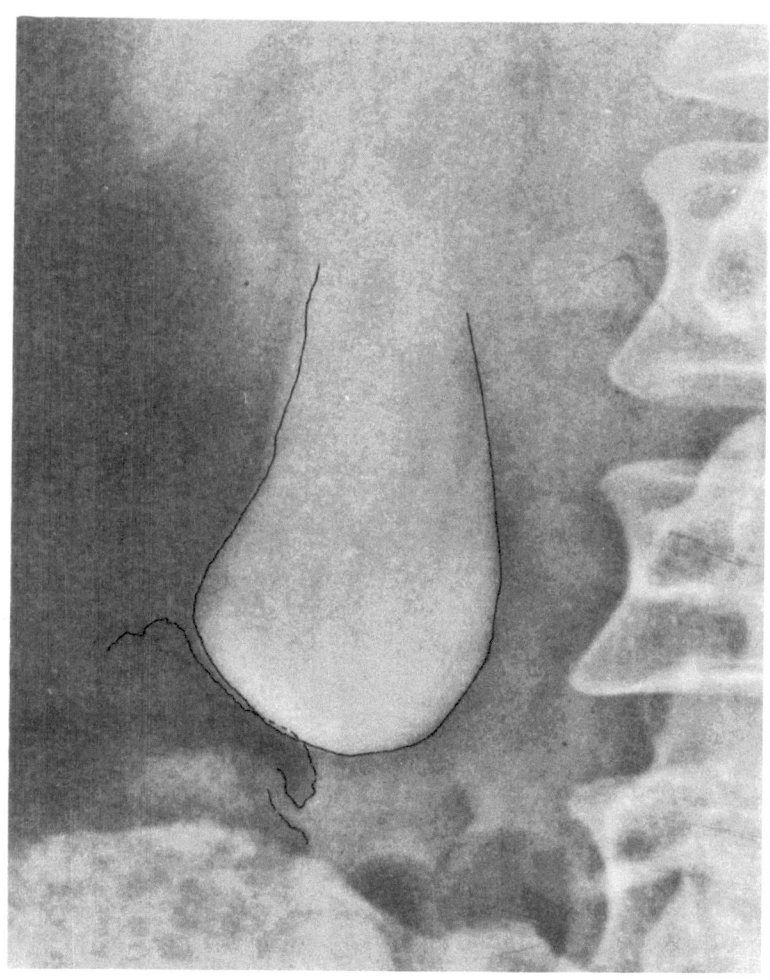

1. Good concentration.
2. Pseudo Rokitansky-
   Aschoff Sinus.
   Misinterpretation.

IV. SOME ROENTGENDIAGNOSTIC SUGGESTIONS

Roentgendiagnosis of degenerative conditions of the gallbladder wall does not depend on sophisticated methods of investigation which are unusual in the day to day practice of the radiologist.

It goes almost without saying that the greatest possible care must be taken in radiological investigation of the gallbladder, because the only method capable of demonstrating the hyperplastic cholecystoses is roentgendiagnosis. It is therefore desirable to give attention to some aspects of radiological gallbladder investigation in so far as they are of importance in diagnosing the cholecystoses.

Contrast medium

In principle, it makes no difference whether the iodine-containing contrast medium is given orally or intravenously.

Intravenous administration is preferred when there are indefinite findings based on the oral cholecystogram, or if there is a possible lack of absorption from the gastrointestinal tract.

Exposure technique

Radiographs are made utilizing both fluoroscopic spot films and conventional films. Optimal contrast necessitates utilizing the lowest possible KV. In obese and older patients this can present problems, so that compression films and adequate coning have to be used. During fluoroscopic examination, one must remember that, in making spot-exposures, a grid need not necessarily be used. This can lead to considerable improvement in contrast.

Only as a last resort should increased kilovoltage be applied.

It is often sufficient to make a small number of exposures with the patient in erect and supine position. Administration of a contraction meal or intravenous injection of cholecystokinin (see page 119) is necessary for a better demonstration of Rokitansky-Aschoff sinuses and the degree of gallbladder contraction (28). It is important that the exposures be made by the same examiner, who will be on the alert to notice less obvious discrepancies.

Functional gallbladder investigation

When, despite negative findings on conventional X-ray films, suspicion of the existence of a cholecystosis still remains, it is necessary to extend the investigation to what is known as functional intravenous cholangiogram. This entails investigation of the gallbladder exclusively in accordance with functional criteria known as the 'hyperfunction-complex', also called (21) 'the triad of Jutras':

1. Hyperconcentration of the contrast material as a result of mucosal hyperplasia. Increase in the number of mucosal cell elements is believed to result in a more marked degree of concentration of the contrast medium.
2. Hyperexcitability of the gallbladder due to neuromatosis which is frequently combined with other forms of cholecystosis. This manifests itself in a more rapid reaction to a fatty meal and can occur within a few minutes after administration.
3. Hyperexcretion: more powerful emptying of the gallbladder due to the hyperplastic muscularis. In some cases the gallbladder might even be totally evacuated.

This way of demonstrating degenerative conditions of the gallbladder wall is purely functional, the function of the gallbladder being examined in the absence of other, more obvious morphological criteria. A more or less standarised method of administration for the contrast medium, i.e. intravenously, should take preference over the oral route.

In general, films may be taken at 5 minute intervals both before and after administration of the fatty meal. According to the publication of Jutras et al. (33), this method is specially suited for demonstrating adenomyomatosis. But due to the lack of objective criteria, this method of investigation has not yet been generally accepted.

Follow-up studies

If the changes on the X-ray films are too scanty for diagnosis of a gallbladder wall degeneration, studies must be repeated at monthly or yearly intervals, because it has often been shown that these changes only become visible with time (7).

CLINICAL ASPECTS

V. ETIOLOGY AND FREQUENCY

The three types described here are merely a selection of cholecystoses as proposed by Jutras (see table), but are relatively the easiest to diagnose roentgenologically and the most common types.

Etiological factors are poorly understood. Agreement, however, exists about their being non-malignant and mostly non-infectious. The incidence is rather varied and is mostly based on necropsy (11, 24) and cholecystogram studies (12, 34).

V.1 Hyalinocalcinosis

The least frequent of the cholecystoses seems to be the hyalinocalcinosis as no report − to our knowledge − states the frequency of this condition. Most handbooks on gastroenterology mention the condition as an incidental finding in upper abdominal roentgenology. It is suggested (15) that it is mostly concomitant with chronic cholecystitis, which almost invariably develops in association with gallstones. Recurrent bouts of inflammation cause the wall of the gallbladder to become thickened, opacified and calcified. Histological inspection of the chronically inflamed gallbladder, confirms the presence of fibrous tissue as the cause of this thickening. Areas of mucosal ulceration are often found, probably as the result of trauma from stones in the lumen. Endarteriitis obliterans is frequently encountered in the vessels of the gallbladder wall (46).

V.2 Cholesterolosis

As in other forms of cholecystoses the frequency of this particular type is mostly based on retrospective necropsy and cholecystogram studies. In a series of 1062 cholecystectomies 167 cholecystoses were found of which 90 were cholesterosis (53.8%) (5). Autopsy studies reveal frequencies ranging from 12.5 tot 38.5% (24). In this condition also concomitant

Hyperplastic cholecystoses

I.	*Cholesterolosis*	synonyms
	A. Diffuse type (disseminated micro-nodules)	Strawberry gallbladder cholesterosis lipoid cholecystitis
	B. Polypoid type	pedunculated polyp: solitary or multiple sessile polyp
II.	*Adenomyomatosis*	
	A. Generalized type	cholecystitis glandularis proliferans
	B. Segmental type	cystic cholecystitis intramural diverticulosis pneumocholecyst with intramural bullae parietal calculi
	C. Localized type	adenomyoma adenoma adenofibromyoma epithelioma myoepithelial anomaly
III.	*Superficial neuromatosis*	
IV.	*Deep neuromatosis*	
V.	*Elastosis*	
VI.	*Lipomatosis*	
VII.	*Interstitial fibromatosis*	
VIII.	*Pericholecystic fibromatosis*	
IX.	*Hyalinocalcinosis*	porcelain gallbladder calcified gallbladder calcifying cholecystitis

After: Jutras, J.A., Hyperplastic Cholecystosis; *Amer. J. Roentgenol.*, 1960, *83*, 795.

cholelithiasis is to be found. Findings range from 71.2% (5) to only 10% (24). Female-male sex prevalence ratios range from 4.4:1 to 1:1 (5, 24, 4). Any frequency based on these kind of studies may be found and it is obvious that hardly any clinical significance can exist. Etiologically this condition is again non-inflammatory.

The wall of the gallbladder forms pseudopolyps protruding into the gallbladder lumen which consist of foamy histiocytes containing esters of cholesterol and an outer layer of columnar epithelium (9). From the outside they may – during operation – appear as yellow excrescencies arising on a small pedicle from a mucosa which is usually otherwise normal. Sometimes there is a diffuse speckling of the mucosa with small lipid accumulations which gives rise to its name of 'strawberry gallbladder'. Occasionally these polyps may be detached from their site of origin and possibly become a source of stone nucleus.

Inflammation is rarely the cause of this condition, but may be present as a secundary phenomenon. Hyperplasia of neural tissue has been found in histopathological investigations (18) and it was therefore called neurogenous cholecystopathy. Other investigators (17) considered disturbances in cholesterol metabolism the primary factor and in their concept the gallbladder plays a completely passive role. In relative contradiction to this is the observation that in a series of 269 cases of cholesterosis no evidence of hypercholesterolaemia was found (42).

The most recent and up till now most accepted theory is the hyperexcitability, hyperconcentration and hypersecretion syndrome proposed by Jutras.

V.3 Adenomyomatosis

The frequency of this condition, based on prospective studies of cholecystograms, is about 5% (19, 33). It should be mentioned however, that this frequency is based on studies performed by investigators looking for the condition. In this respect it is worthwhile mentioning, that in a retrospective study of 4000 necropsies a group of investigators found only 0.4% cases of adenomyomatosis, but prospectively they found 7% in 200 (11).

As with cholelithiasis it is more frequent in females than in males. Ratios ranging from 3:1 to 3:2 (5, 12, 33, 34). Etiologically several factors have been investigated and of these the mechanism proposed by Jutras seems the most likely. As a consequence of increased pressure within the gallbladder (the nature of which is still under discussion, although several authors have presented evidence for the existence of a hypersensitivity to cholecystokinin in several of these cases (13, 26)), hyperplasia of all structures of the wall of the gallbladder occurs in which small diverticular cysts develop, named after their discoverers the Rokitansky-Aschoff sinuses (R.A.S.) (6, 41). As a result of this hyperplasia hypersecretion from the mucosa occurs which may lead to branching and formation of multisaccular structures out of the sinuses and even to stricture of the neck of the sinus (12) and sometimes small concrements may be found in the neck (2). Whether these changes are due only to increased pressure within the gallbladder (2, 14, 33) is by no means certain and a recent observation seems here to be of interest (38).

A patient has been described in whom, in connection with a hiatal hernia and gastro-oesophageal reflux, a spastic area of muscular hypertrophy was found in which segmental intramural diverticula were seen and the oesophagus was − as is the gallbladder − lined with columnar epithelium. The question arises whether these diverticula are etiologically comparable with R.A.S.

Inflammation has long been encountered in most cases, but since the thirties opinions have changed from definitely inflammatory (35), via probably inflammatory (2) to non-inflammatory (43) and a recent study suggests inflammation as being secundary to R.A.S. (36). The views of the relationship between cholelithiasis and adenomyomatosis have similarly changed (5) and relatively recent studies have confirmed the non-calculous nature of the condition (10).

Congenital or developmental anomalies are also suggested, but R.A.S. have not been encountered in children (35).

Perhaps the most important conclusion may be drawn from a follow-up study of 196 cases of adenomyomatosis for 15 years in which no signs of malignancy were found (16).

VI. CLINICAL SYMPTOMATOLOGY

The relationships between cholecystoses and the clinical syndrome are scantily documented. In the literature some case reports are to be found (7, 22, 23, 45). Restrospective studies are available on adenomyomatosis and cholesterolosis. In a series of 21 cases of adenomyomatosis 8 were found to have biliary symptoms (19).

In a series of 269 cases of proven cholesterolosis (42) the following symptoms were found: pain in 96%, food intolerance (specially fat) in 92%, vomiting in 61% and colic in 57%. In another series of 125 cases (4) pain was reported in 77.8%, food intolerance in 68.6%, vomiting in 14.4% and colic in 8.8% while 4% were symptom free.

The wide variety in symptomatology of biliary diseases is well known and 'classic' symptoms are now scarcely encountered, while on the other hand the differential diagnosis may be elaborate. A study of complaints in patients with proven cholelithiasis or nephrolithiasis has shown a rather confused picture with regard to the nature and severity of colic (20). Besides this it should be mentioned, that clinical reports are hampered by the infamiliarity of most clinicians with the conditions and one might suppose that at least in quite a few cases of post or propter proven cholecystoses the indication for the removal of the gallbladder may well have been initiated rather by despair on the part of the clinician than by objective criteria.

More elaborate clinical investigations and more experimental evidence are needed to put the roentgenological findings into their proper clinical place. One way to diagnose these conditions more accurately is the introduction of cholecystokinin cholecystography (13, 26). Cholecysto-kinin (C.C.K.) has a direct effect on the gallbladder muscle as has been shown in studies in guinea pigs (47) and man (29). The contraction of the gallbladder following the infusion of C.C.K. is not altered by any autonomic blockade (29) and seems – therefore – to exert its effect directly. In a group of 7 patients with right upper quadrant abdominal pains after meals in which no gallstones were demonstrated, the infusion of C.C.K. provoked pain in these patients and during cholecystography an impaired gallbladder evacuation due to a partial cystic duct obstruction was seen (cystic duct syndrome) (13). In a well documented series of 42 cases with acalculous biliary tract symptoms it was possible to differentiate between cystic duct syndrome, partial obstruction at the sphincter of Oddi and hyperplastic cholecystoses by using the C.C.K. cholecystography. In hyperplastic cholecystoses hypercontraction of the gallbladder was seen (26).

VII. THERAPY

It is hardly surprising that therapy of these cholecystoses is as variable as the clinical picture. As the condition has proved to be not premalignant, a tendency to medical treatment is obvious and justified.

As fat intolerance is a dominant complaint, dietary restriction of fat is essential. Further spasmodics can be of use (30). Depending on the severity of the symptoms cholecystectomy should be considered although the benefit of this surgical intervention is not yet firmly established. In his study of 269 cases Salmenkivi (42) demonstrated in the follow-up complete recovery in 69%, persistent distress in 18% and no benefit in 12%. In another series (5) these percentages were respectively 53%, 34% and 14%. In a series of 8 cases of adenomyomatosis 100% recovery following surgery has been reported (19, 32). These figures are consistent with the observation, that removal of the symptomatic acalculous gallbladder·results in good relief of symptoms in only 64% (25). It has been suggested (31), that the presence of R.A.S. is an indication for cholecystectomy since the R.A.S. sometimes contain stones which may erode the mucosa and therefore may either be a source of stone formation, or a source of peritonitis due to penetration of the gallbladder wall.

When cholecystectomy should be performed it is necessary – especially in cases of cholesterosis – that the content of the gallbladder is inspected during operation to establish the diagnosis (42). In addition one should perform the cholecystectomy in such a way, that histopathological studies are possible. Especially in the fundal type of adenomyomatosis the surgeon should refrain from clipping the gallbladder.

In summary, the cholecystoses are of clinical importance, although conviction here is not yet general. It is essential to look for these conditions in patients with complaints directed to the biliary system for which no other source can be found.

Treatment is mainly dependent on the severity of symptoms and cholecystectomy is in certain cases justified. Medical treatment with low fat content diets and spasmodics is indicated in those patients whose symptoms are mild.

ACKNOWLEDGEMENTS

We are indebted to many colleagues who made the presentation of this collection of radiographs possible. Especially we would like to thank G.J. Van Andel, M.D. and co-workers (Diaconessenhuis, Eindhoven), who willingly offered a collection of radiographs without which publication of this book hardly had been possible. Besides we are thankfull to those who taught us and stimulated us in studying the diagnostics of gallbladder diseases and specially the degenerative abnormalities. In this we may name Professor C.B.A.J. Puijlaert, M.D., Professor A.C. Klinkhamer, M.D. and O.J. ten Thije, M.D.

                                                        J.H.J. Ruijs
                                                        S.G.Th. Hulst

REFERENCES

1. Aguirre, J.R., Boher, R.O. and Gurdieb, S., Hyperplastic cholecystoses; a new contribution to the Unitarian Theory. *Amer. J. Roentgenol.* 1969,*107*, 1.
2. Akerlund, A. and Rudhe, U., Intramural small-cystic diverticulosis of the gallbladder. *Acta Radiol.* 1950, *33*, 147.
3. Alcorn, F.S. and Frank, R.J., Rokitansky-Aschoff sinuses as a presumptive X-ray sign of gallbladder disease. *Arch. Surg.* 1957,*74*, 500.
4. Arianoff, A.A., *Les cholecystoses.* Arscia/Maloine, Paris 1961.
5. Arianoff, A.A., Henrard, E.H. and Van Dessel, A., Considerations radiologiques et cliniques sur les cholecystoses. *J. belge Radiol.* 1962,*45*, 97.
6. Aschoff, K.A.L. Bemerkungen zur pathologischen Anatomie der Cholelithiasis und Cholecystitis. *Verh. dtsch. path. Ges.* 1905,*9*, 41.
7. Bender, J., Van Andel, G.J. en Hoefsloot, F.A.M., De adenomyomatose van de galblaas. *Ned. T. Geneesk.*, 1974,*118*, 1324.
8. Berk, R.N. and Loeb, P.M., Pharmacology and Physiology of the Biliary Radiographic Contrast Materials, Seminars in Roentgenology, 1976, *XI*, 147.
9. Bevan, G., Tumours of the gallbladder. *Clinics in Gastroenterology,* 1973,*2*, 175.
10. Bevan, G., Acalculous adenomyomatosis of the gallbladder. *Gut*, 1970,*2*, 1029.
11. Bricker, D.L. and Halpert, B., Adenomyoma of the gallbladder. *Surgery*, 1963,*53*, 615.
12. Colquhoun, J., Adenomyomatosis of the gallbladder (intramural diverticulosis). *Brit. J. Radiol*, 1961,*34*, 101.
13. Cozzolino, H.J., Goldstein, F., Greening, R.R. and Wirts, C.W., The cystic duct syndrome. *J. Amer. med. Ass.*, 1963,*185*, 920.
14. Culver, G.J., Berens, D.L. and Bean, B.C., Relationship of stenosis to Rokitansky-Aschoff sinuses of the gallbladder. *Amer. J. Roentgenol.* 1957,*7*, 47.
15. Dawson, J.L., Cholecystitis and cholecystectomy. *Clinics in Gastroenterology,* 1973,*2*, 85.
16. Eelkema, H.H., Hodgson, J.R., and Stauffer, M.H., Fifteen year follow-up of polypoid lesions of the gallbladder diagnosed by cholecystography. *Gastroenterology,* 1962,*42*, 144.
17. Feldman, M., Smith, M. and Warner, C.G., Die hepatische Grundlage der Gallenblasen-Cholesterose: Eine neue Auffassung über deren Ätiologie. Read for the IInd World Congress of Gastroenterology, München, 1962.
18. Feyrter, F., Zur Pathogenese der sog. Stippchengallenblase. *Langenbeck Arch. Klin. Chir.* 1958,*290*, 86.
19. Fotopoulos, J.P. and Crampton, A.R., Adenomyomatosis of the gallbladder *Med. Clinics North America*, 1964,*48*, 9.
20. French, E.B. and Robb, W.A.T. Biliary and renal colic. *Brit. med. J.* 1963,*2*, 135.
21. Frommhold, W. and Lagemann, K., Die Adenomyomatose der Gallenblase. *Fortsch. Röntgenstr.* 1971,*115*, 464.
22. Geldof, W.Ch.P., Een patiënte met een zandlopergalblaas. *Ned. T. Geneesk.* 1967,*111*, 1463.
23. Geldof, W.Ch.P. and Scheffer, E., Een patiënte met een zandlopergalblaas met divertikels van Rokitansky-Aschoff. *Ned. T. Geneesk.* 1969,*113*, 1648.
24. Gérolami, A., Tumeurs bénignes et formations pseudo-tumorales des voies biliaires. In: *Foie, Pancréas, Voies biliaires.* Ed. J.-P. Benhamou and H. Sarles, Pathologie Médicale No. 5, Flammarion médicine sciences. Paris. 1972, 166.
25. Glenn, F. and Mannix, H. Jr., The acalculous gallbladder. *Ann. Surg.* 1956,*144*, 670.

26. Goldstein, F., Grunt, R. and Margulis, M., Cholecystokinin Cholecystography in the differential diagnosis of acalculous gallbladder disease. *Amer. J. dig. Dis.* 1974,*19*, 835.
27. Halpert, B. Morpholological studies on the gallbladder. I. A note on developmental and macroscopic structure of normal human gallbladder. *Bull. Johns. Hopk. Hosp.*, 1927,*40*, 390.
28. Harvey, I.C., Myo Thwe and Low-Beer, T.S., The value of the fatty meal in oral cholecystography. *Clin. Radiol.* 1976,*27*, 117.
29. Harvey, R.F., Hormonal control of gastrointestinal motility. *Amer. J. dig. Dis.* 1975,*20*, 523.
30. Heald, R.J., Adenomyomatosis as a source of error in the diagnosis of gallbladder disease. *Brit. J. Surg.* 1970,*57*, 353.
31. Hepp, J., Vésicule fraise et cholécystite avec sinus de Rokitansky. *Actualités hépato-gastroentérologiques de l'Hôtel-Dieu,* Paris, Masson et Cie, 1958.
32. Jacobs, L.A., De Meester, T.R., Eggleston, J.C., Magulies, S.I. and Zuidema, G.D., Hyperplastic cholecystoses. *Arch. Surg.* 1972,*104*, 193.
33. Jutras, J.A., Longtin, J.M. and Lévesque, H.P., Hyperplastic cholecystoses. *Amer. J. Roentgenol.* 1960,*83*, 795.
34. Jutras, J.A. and Lévesque, H.P., Adenomyoma and adenomyomatosis of the gallbladder. *Radiol. Clin. North Amer.* 1966,*4*, 483.
35. King, E.S.J. and MacCallum, P., Cholecystitis glandularis proliferans (cystica). *Brit. J. Surg.* 1931,*19*, 310.
36. LeQuesne, L.P. and Ranger, I., Cholecystitis glandularis proliferans. *Brit. J. Surg.*, 1957,*44*, 447.
37. March, H.C., Visualization of the Rokitansky-Aschoff sinuses of the gallbladder during cholecystography. *Amer. J. Roentgenol.* 1948,*59*, 197.
38. Mendl, K., Montgomery, R.D. and Stephenson, S.F., Segmental intramural diverticulosis associated with and confined to a spastic area of muscular hypertrophy in a columnar lined oesophagus. *Clin. Radiol.* 1973,*24*, 440.
39. Ochsner, S.F., Adenomyoma of the gallbladder. *Amer. J. Roentgenol.* 1962,*88*, 778.
40. Robertsson, H.E., and Ferguson, W.J., The diverticula (Luschka's crypts) of the gallbladder. *Arch. Pathol.* 1946,*40*, 312.
41. Rokitansky, C. von, In: *Handbuch der Speziellen Pathologischen Anatomie.* 1842, II, 374. Braumüller & Seidel, Wien.
42. Salmenkivi, K., Cholesterosis of the gallbladder. *Acta chirugica scand.* 1964, suppl. 324.
43. Selzer, D.W., Dockerty, M.B., Stauffer, M.H. and Priestly, J.T., Papillomas (so-called) in the non-calculous gallbladder. *Amer. J. Surg.* 1962,*103*, 472.
44. Sutherland, L.R., Small adenomyoma of the gallbladder. *Glasgow med. J.*, 1898,*50*, 216.
45. Valberg, L.S., Jabbari, M., Kerr, J.W., Curtis, A.C., Ramchard, S. and Prentice, R.S.A., Biliary pain in young women in the absence of gallstones. *Gastroenterology,* 1971,*60*, 1020.
46. Varay, A., Les cholecystoses. *Rev. Prat.* 1971,*21*, 67.
47. Yau, W.M., Makhlouf, G.M., Edwards, L.E. and Farra, J.T. Mode of action of cholecystokinin and related peptides on gallbladder muscle. *Gastroenterology,* 1973,*65*, 451.

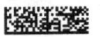